WHAT O̲

Laurie is a successful graduate of multiple Fitness, Nutrition, and Health Certifications offered here at the Cooper Institute, Dallas, Texas. I was one of her instructors for many of the topics and got to know Laurie more personally. This freedom and fitness devotional is a work of love from Laurie. Because she herself had to overcome excessive weight gain and the emotional bruises that led to such behaviors, Laurie is very compassionate, but also very savvy about navigating the ups and downs and potential pitfalls that can challenge even the most determined person. Laurie not only has a good command of health and fitness information but she is also a mature, devoted Christian. Her knowledge of the Word of God comes alive as we are motivated by the daily devotionals to guide our way spirit, soul, and body.

—Karyn Hughes, M.Ed. in Kinesiology,
Associate Director of Education,
The Cooper Institute, Dallas, Texas

Laurie has great insight into the spirit, soul and body connection in relation to health and fitness. This book motivates, inspires and provides effective tools for personal transformation as it reveals the truths of success for personal development. Let Laurie coach you on a journey to becoming fit and free.

—Bruce and Lisa Barlean,
Barlean's Organic Oils

Laurie's devotional offers the reader quite a bit of information on their journey to reach their dietary and fitness goals. In particular, the use of powerful quotations of the Word of God acts as THE foundation from which all steps are taken. Each chapter presents a relevant biblical perspective which gives the reader a sense of purpose as they progress. People fail in achieving their goals purely from broken focus, and this aspect of Laurie's book, when used daily as intended, will keep the believer on target to hit those goals. In Revelation 12:11 we are taught to defeat the enemy by "the blood of the Lamb, and the word of our testimony". Laurie uses her awesome testimony to advantage. Chapters 16, 21, 27, and 29 were specifically POWERFUL and full of comprehension...Laurie has offered us a working knowledge of God's Word in order to defeat the enemy on our way to accomplishing our goals. Bring on more of that Laurie!!!

—John Heart, 2013 Mr. America

As a former Biggest Loser Contestant that has started a health ministry, I was moved, touched, and excited by the use of scriptural truths in the journey towards health. Laurie guides the reader on the journey towards health inciting change and action within them. I think this devotional could be the difference maker in a personal journey towards a balanced lifestyle of faith and fitness.

—Austin Andrews,
Cofounder of RetroFit Ministries
Former Contestant on NBC's
The Biggest Loser, Season 11.

One of the most powerful sermon series and events that Northwood Church has ever had was the "Losing IT" series and the Fit for Freedom Challenge that followed. I'd like to says I came up with the idea–but I didn't. Laurie came up with the concept, invited former contestants from *The Biggest Loser* to be our guest speakers and implemented the wellness program–it was HUGE! I personally benefited from it and I started on a journey that I'm currently continuing. This devotional is a result of her efforts and is not just about weight loss, but spiritual and emotional health as well. Our church numerically grew during this period as a result of this wellness program and outreach. Pastor friends, I encourage you to consider providing an opportunity like this in your church and practice it in your own life as well .

—Pastor Bob Roberts
Northwood Church, Keller, Texas
Author of *Bold as Love*

Laurie has written an excellent devotional focusing on physical fitness. She stresses the steps necessary in achieving a physically healthy life.

Some key points are: taking responsibility, identifying the giants that try to control your life, trusting God by learning who we are and what power is available to us as believers and taking action because all the great intentions and plans are worthless and will accomplish nothing if we don't take action.

These are just a few of the steps spelled out in Laurie's devotional. But they all add up to healing. Laurie's use of Scripture and prayer for each day stresses the most important element of healing. That element is our communication with God and knowing His will for our lives. The devotional has added value for me as a Licensed Professional Counselor. Each of the steps used parallels healing of emotional problems as well. I find that Laurie's devotional is useful in healing no matter what the issue or addiction may be.

—Dwayne Collins, MA, LCP,
Heart Change Ministry, LP,
Flower Mound, Texas

My wife and family have know Laurie, her parents and family for over 30 years. What a blessing and inspiration she has been to so many!

I know that anyone would benefit and grow closer to The Lord by reading and adhering to the principles in this book. This is more than a weight-loss devotional. You might call it a sin-loss, apathy-loss, low self esteem-loss, inferiority-loss, and so much more "loss" book. Make no mistake about it though, what you will gain is so much better than what you will lose. Laurie teaches spiritual fitness as the true way to lasting physical fitness. This is not about abstract theory but concrete principles confirmed with inspiring testimonies that follow each daily devotion.

Laurie has put a lot of thought, hard work, personal transparency, and passion into this "labor of love". I have been greatly blessed by it and I know you will too.

—Pastor Michael W. Williams,
International Outreach Church,
Wills Point, Texas

Laurie's true gifts shine through each and every page of this book. For anyone who is struggling with health and weight issues and addictions, Laurie's experience, this book and what the Word of God says about it have everything you need to start on your own journey of healing and health from the inside out!

—Charline Bucher, Time As This, Inc.,
Team Beach Body Coach &
Grand Prize Winner

Laurie is so transparent. Her genuinely sweet spirit shines through on the pages of this book, and it is truly her heart's greatest desire to help others gain victory over their health. Her incredible testimony and the testimonies of others that she shares are so encouraging. Every reader will find one or more that they can relate to; connect with. This devotional will change your thinking and it will change you, if you will allow it to. If you're still busy licking old wounds and not ready for change then do not begin reading this devotional. However, if you are ready to begin experiencing all that God has for you–life to the fullest, then work through this devotional and perform each exercise that Laurie provides. She has Holy Spirit revealed insights and instruction that will provide you with hope, healing, and most of all, the abundant life that Christ has promised to each of us. And the greatest part is that it is contagious: as you find help and experience victory in your own life you will become empowered to help others. It is all part of God's master plan to bless us abundantly so that we can abundantly bless those around us. Make a commitment for the next 30 days to read this book of daily devotions and you will be well on your way to regaining your health – body, mind and spirit.

—Denise McDonald
Certified Nutritional Counselor
Nourshing Your Body, LLC

I have thoroughly enjoyed reading *Fit for Freedom*. As a previous "Loser" and now personal trainer, I understand that losing weight is much more than eating right and exercise. It's about getting to the root of the problem and learning how to overcome those issues. For those people that are sincerely trying to make a change and don't know where to start, this devotional is a great guide to begin breaking through those emotional barriers.

—Elizabeth Ruiz
Former Finalist on NBC's
The Biggest Loser, Season 10

As a Pastor and person that has struggled with food addiction my entire life I HIGHLY recommend this devotional to folks that desire to be fit spirit, soul, and body. The topics and scripture shared are doctrinally sound and relevant to all regardless of where they are on their fitness journey. My only complaint is that this amazing tool was not available for me 2 years ago when I began my own personal journey!

—Pastor Chris Pedersen, Children's Pastor,
Northstar Christian Center,
Columbia, SC

Working to improve physical fitness without addressing your spiritual struggles sets the stage for certain failure. Graves knows this, she has experienced it first hand and her commitment to help others avoid this unintended but most common type of self-sabotage is the defining difference in *Fit for Freedom*. She fills each devotional-length chapter with Bible-based guidance and encouraging accounts of others who have struggled and overcome. The result is a unique 30-day nurturing she has prayerfully crafted, which gives you easy-to-understand instruction blended with spirit-building inspiration. We need more personal trainers to connect faith and fitness the way Laurie has done.

—Brad Bloom,
Publisher Faith & Fitness Magazine
www.faithandfitness.net

FIT FOR FREEDOM

FIT FOR FREEDOM
HEALING FOR YOUR BODY, MIND, AND SPIRIT

BY LAURIE GRAVES

With former contestants from
NBC's The Biggest Loser and
ABC's Extreme Weight Loss

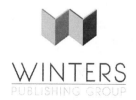

WINTERS
PUBLISHING GROUP

Published by Winters Publishing
2448 E. 81st St.
Suite #4802
Tulsa, OK 74137

Book Design Copyright 2014 by Winters Publishing. All rights reserved.
Cover design by Aaron Thompkins
Interior design by Caypeeline Casas

Published in the United States of America

ISBN: 978-1-63063-066-9
Health & Fitness / Diet & Nutrition
14.01.28

DEDICATION

To my beautiful girls Haley and Sophia,
you are loved and cherished.

DISCLAIMER

The Biggest Loser and *Extreme Weight Loss* are not associated with this book in any way or the information within.

This book is meant to be a guide in spiritual and physical wellness. It has been carefully researched to provide the most accurate and helpful information; however, it should not be used as a replacement to professional medical advice. Always consult your doctor or healthcare provider before beginning any health or wellness program.

ACKNOWLEDGEMENTS

Many thanks to Mr. Tom Winters and Winters Publishing Group for believing in the message of this book and allowing me the opportunity to see a dream fulfilled.

Dr. Robert Tate, I appreciate your guidance and encouragement that let me know I was on the right track with this project. You will never know how much it meant to me to hear your own personal story of weight loss and transformation. Thank you for sharing that with me. I will always remember the day I signed my contract as the day God moved heaven and earth AND Paula Dean to get me in the production line. Thank you for being a part of my miracle.

To my former weight loss reality show friends: Aaron Thompkins, Danny Cahill, Sean Algaier, Julie Hadden, Ken Andrews, Corey Pinkerton, and Staci Birdwell, thank you for sharing your personal experiences to enhance the teachings in this book. I believe that your transparency will be the catalyst for many to find the courage to start their journey. I appreciate your willingness to help with this project; it has been a pleasure working with all of you.

Pastor Bob Roberts, thank you for allowing me to write the outline for the 2012 sermon series entitled, *Losing IT.* Because you believed in the idea of a health and wellness series and allowed me to lead the Fit for Freedom Challenge at Northwood Church, this book was conceptualized and written. I appreciate you supporting my ministry to Northwood and beyond.

Fit for Freedom participants, YOU ROCK! You gave it your all, you learned, worked hard, and you reaped blessings in your spirit, soul, and body. Most of you lost weight, inches, and habits but even more importantly, all of you lost emotional baggage that was inhibiting you from moving forward in weight loss and in life. Thank you for trusting me to teach you and lead you on the journey that I personally had to go through to walk toward my own freedom. I am honored that you lent me your stories to help others who have picked up this book to start their own journey toward healthy living.

Pastor John Osteen, you're dancing with the angels, but I will never forget the impact you had on my life. As a young girl I saw you and Sister Dodie love unconditionally, I heard you speak the uncompromised Word of God, I saw you pray for the sick, and saw God heal and deliver them. Because of my family's time at Lakewood Church, I believe I was set up to walk through the trials I've been through and cling to Him knowing that by faith I would come out on top. Because of your teachings, I believe that my spirit was set up to recall and relay the concepts in this devotional. Thank you for always standing firm in what you believed even when it went against popular opinion.

Mom and Dad, thank you for continuing the heritage of faith in our home. Thank you for the investment of faith and healing teaching that you poured into our family.

Shirita Schneider, my editor extraordinaire, without you, who knows what may have happened?! I appreciate your effort to get my writing straightened up and worthy of reading. Thank you for your diligence to this undertaking. Your kind words and encouragement throughout the writing and editing process were a blessing from Heaven. There is truly no one like you!

Paul Schneider, it was your work that got me noticed! From your great marketing suggestions and eye catching graphics, you are a true professional. Thank you for your support and for investing into this project and helping me land the big fish.

Dearest Michael, my sweet husband and friend, thank you for holding my hand and telling me that I could succeed in this profession and ministry. You'll never know how much it has meant to have you alongside of me, supporting me, and speaking words of life over me and this project. Your blessings of encouragement as I prepared the material and put it all together has been simply priceless. Baby, you're the *best*!

CONTENTS

FOREWORD

by Danny Cahill, *The Biggest Loser* Winner, Season 8

When you weigh 460 pounds and every step feels like it could be your last, you're desperate. I know I was. I prayed about the situation—and so did my wife, Darci, and I decided to try out for *The Biggest Loser*! Well, out of hundreds of thousands of entrants, I made one of 16 spots on the show. As I left my family behind for the Biggest Loser ranch, I was scared to death! I didn't know what to expect, but I did know one thing: God had given me this opportunity and I was going to give it my all! Six and a half months later I weighed in at the Season 8 finale, and had lost 239 pounds! I had become the Biggest Loser EVER in the history of the show! Not only that, but my wife had lost 70 pounds on her own! Our lives had changed for good! Or so I thought.

Two years after the finale of *The Biggest Loser*, I had kept the weight off. I became a professional motivational speaker and was speaking all over the United States, and even overseas, for companies, churches, organizations and charities. While speaking at a retreat in Georgia, I received the news that my father had unexpectedly passed away. I was in shock. The flight home was the longest flight I had ever taken in my life. It seemed to take forever! On the layover home, I went into a restaurant and ordered food. I ate it, but didn't feel satisfied. I ordered more and ate a second portion.

I returned home to be with my family. People brought us meals out of love, and I ate them! We buried my father, and over the next 45 days I quickly gained 35 pounds. My wife let me mourn, but when she saw I was falling back into my addiction, she confronted me. Darci said, "Babe, I love you, and I know it's been hard, but you've got to stop." I thought after winning the eighth season of *The Biggest Loser*, I had conquered my addiction—but all it took was a difficult time in my life to fall right back into that trap—the trap of nothing being enough to fill that empty hole I felt in my heart. Instead of turning to God, I turned back to food.

Losing the weight for a second time has proven a struggle. I still need to lose 20 pounds, and it seems harder than shedding the 239 pounds I lost on the show! But I knew that going back to an extreme method of weight loss would not solve my problem. It would only be a matter of time until another stressful situation arose and I would try to deal with it by overeating. A true lifestyle change was the only thing that would work.

When I met Laurie Graves, she was training a friend of mine for season 10 of *The Biggest Loser*. She had something about her that impressed me. I'd never seen her train before, but when she talked about God and the love He has for us, I knew that her method of training was bigger than simply telling someone what to do and what to eat. She was using God's love, as well as sound training, to change the lives of those around her. When Laurie asked me to write the foreword for her book, I didn't hesitate. Her heart for people is big; so big that she that she has spent a lot of time and invested much of her own money into changing people's lives. She truly has a heart for people and for our Lord.

Laurie is an amazing inspiration to so many people. Through her past experiences and trials, she has turned what was meant to harm her into a path of good for the people she meets. I know some of those whom she has trained physically, and they are fitter and stronger than ever. But most importantly, the mental and spiritual aspects of her beliefs are an incredible foundation for those wishing to change their lives and follow the path that God has for them. I have read Laurie's devotional and have been inspired to begin a new journey for myself. I believe that everyone who reads it will find hope and inspiration in their walk with the Lord on their journey to a better life.

Danny Cahill
Winner of *The Biggest Loser*
International Motivational/Inspirational Speaker
Author of *Losing Big* and *Lose Your Quit*
www.TheDannyCahill.com

INTRODUCTION

When I was young, my family and I lived in Spokane, Washington. It's a beautiful part of the country, just 30 miles south of the Canadian border. We had a fairly active lifestyle there in the great Northwest. My parents took us hiking with friends, we played in the snow, and camped—all typical activities for that area. My mom planted her own garden and we would go to nearby orchards to pick apples and pears—fruit which we not only ate just off the tree, but also canned to enjoy in the colder fall and winter months. Because we raised or picked much of the food we ate, we enjoyed a healthy diet that included lots of fresh organic fruits and vegetables.

When I was 11, my dad took a job that required a transfer to Houston, Texas. We liked Texas, but the heat and small yard at our new home made it hard to garden. And some of the outdoor activities we participated in were no longer enjoyable in the Texas heat.

Even though it was hot in Texas, there were many good things about Houston. My family became members of Lakewood Church. Lakewood was an exciting church to be a part of! You never knew what God was going to do. Pastor John Osteen had a dynamic way of preaching that kept me on the edge of my seat. Other characteristics that I noticed were the love of God and compassion for others that just flowed out of him.

Every Sunday we would lift our Bibles together and repeat after Pastor John, "This is my Bible. I am what it says I am, I can have what it says I can have, I can do what it says I can do. Today I will be taught the word of God. I boldly confess that my mind is alert, my heart is receptive. I am about to receive the incorruptible, indestructible, ever-living seed of the Word of God. I'll never be the same—never, never, never be the same. In Jesus name, Amen." As I listened to Pastor John preach, the Word became living and alive to me, even at a very young age.

On one Wednesday night in particular I was sitting on the front row waiting for my parents to finish visiting with other congregation members, when out of the corner of my eye I saw a man walk up to Pastor John. I couldn't hear what they were saying, but I could see what was going on. The man was acting strangely, jerking all over the place and his mouth was moving rapidly. Pastor John put his hands on either side of the man's head and I heard him say in a loud voice, "In the name of Jesus, I command you to release this man and set him free!" I got goosebumps. The man struggled, and some men on the other side of the church came over and helped minister. In a matter of minutes, the man sat up and was smiling with tears streaming down his face. He had been set free! Pastor John and the other men were encouraging him and patting him on the back. Seeing my pastor minister deliverance like that made an impression on me that I've never forgotten.

My favorite part of the service was when Pastor John and his wife, Dodie, would stand together and pray for the sick. They flowed in ministry to the ill, the incurable and the downtrodden. Dodie had been healed of cancer many years previously and had a supernatural anointing to pray and minister to the sick. We heard about and saw many people being healed. People drove from all over to come and receive prayer at Lakewood.

There were many things I loved about being at Lakewood: being with my friends, bringing others to church with us, and spending the day on the grounds because it was too far for us to drive home between the Sunday morning and evening services. We got to meet missionaries and preachers from all over the world and be exposed to many different speakers who boldly declared the uncompromised word of God. As I've gotten older, I've realized what a gift it was to grow up in this particular church environment. It was vital to the development of my Christian faith. Seeing miracles gave me faith to trust God and believe that He desires to heal, and that He would heal when I prayed.

In the late 1970's, my dad received a call upon his life to enter full-time ministry and was ordained at Lakewood. He began to travel and preach, and God blessed my dad with an anointing for healing similar to Pastor John's. As a teenager, I saw many miracles through my father's ministry. Deaf ears that could hear once again, blind eyes that could see, cancer and others growths dissolving, and women who were barren being healed and blessed with children.

Being in this atmosphere gave me a strong desire to minister to the sick myself and see them healed. At 14, I received a prophecy that God would anoint my hands, and if I would be obedient to follow His instructions, He would move through me and I would see many healed. I was pretty excited! However, something took me off course.

When I was 15, I fell hard for a youth pastor intern that was working at another church in our city. He was older, handsome, light-hearted, and attentive—the kind of personality I was attracted to. Unfortunately, he wanted me to have sex with him. That was the beginning of a string of sexual relationships.

Because I knew I was being disobedient to God by not keeping my temple pure for my future husband, I became severely depressed. My depression left me feeling that I was helpless to govern my mind and emotions, so I began seeking ways to control my body. I began practicing anorexia and bulimia to make myself as thin as possible. As a result, I became severely malnourished. Malnutrition, in turn, caused extensive medical problems. My bones were breaking for no apparent reason, my hair was falling out, my skin was sallow, and the depression I was experiencing only escalated due to my poor diet and lack of nutrition.

Then for several years, I dated a boy that I thought was "the one." On the day of his college graduation, he called and told me not to come to the ceremony. He told me he didn't want to see me anymore—no further explanation given. I was heartbroken. I thought it was because I wasn't thin enough. Again, I began restricting my food intake to 200 or 300 calories a day so that I could lose weight and win him back. If at any time I felt that I had eaten too much, I would force myself to throw up. After just three months of this behavior, I was 5'10 and weighed

114 pounds. My bones were becoming brittle from mal-nutrition, and I even had some ribs crack when I sneezed.

Then the pendulum swung the other way, and I gained too much weight. I went up and down on the rollercoaster of weight loss and weight gain through-out my 20's. I tried every diet and weight loss program out there. When I was 27, I met a man and fell in love. We were soon married and I had my first child. Over the next few years, I continued on a cycle of increasing weight gain and yo-yo dieting in an effort to control my weight and fit into society's standard of what the female physique should look like. What I thought I should look like and what the enemy told me I needed to look like to be accepted and loved.

In 1999, we were transferred to a small village in The Netherlands. I began to observe the Dutch practic-ing holistic lifestyle concepts. They had a love for nature and the outdoors, healthy eating, smaller portion sizes, a higher fruit and vegetable intake, and moderate daily exercise. Almost everyone I knew in Holland was thin and fit and strong. This was a stark contrast to most of my friends back home. It became apparent to me that the American lifestyle and diet did not support opti-mal health.

Even though I recognized that their way of life was healthier, I didn't eat or exercise like the Dutch. I stayed with my familiar patterns and remained overweight and mostly sedentary. I needed a push to get started on the road to better habits.

That push came when I received a photo in the mail from my mother. The photo was taken at a family reunion back to the US. In this photo were my aunts, my cousins, and all of my cousins' children. Gazing at the picture, I noticed something that was never apparent to me before. There was a legacy of obesity passing through the generations of my family.

On that day, standing in my kitchen, I made a promise to God that I would not let obesity pass on to my daughter. I didn't exactly know what to do, but I started making attempts. Then I unexpectedly became pregnant with my second daughter. Since I was not very many months into my new, healthier lifestyle, I gave up. I used the "pregnancy excuse" and ate enough food for two people. I would eat a healthy salad everyday for lunch, then I would sit on the couch and watch a rerun of *Dallas* (one of the few shows on television in English) while happily munching a Belgian chocolate bar and scarfing down a bag of chips. This got me nowhere, of course, except into increasingly larger pants in a relatively short amount of time.

We returned to the United States soon after I had given birth to my youngest daughter. My weight was at an all-time high of 240 pounds, and I was wearing a size 20. It wasn't just baby weight either—I was a big girl even before I got pregnant. After my pregnancy, the weight just didn't seem to budge.

On my 36th birthday, I finally decided that it was time to get my act together. I was ready to make a change in my life. I gathered the courage to call a fitness trainer who had left a flyer on my door and she said she would come while the baby was sleeping to train me in my garage. I started with small changes and worked up to walking and strength training several times a week. During this time, I lost about 40 pounds.

A year later, I was introduced to another trainer, Kevin Northrop, who was a little more hardcore. Kevin was an excellent fitness coach, who patiently taught me all the fundamentals of weight training. Weekly he would challenge and encourage me, and I got stronger. He thought I could fulfill my dream of competing in figure competitions if I took off more weight. So I turned my body into a shrine, spending three to four hours each day training and preparing my food. I lost a total of 90 pounds and began placing in natural fitness contests. Ultimately, getting in shape for competition became my whole reason for living. I was out of balance, and even though I looked great, another addiction was overtaking me.

You see, I was living a lie. I would eat well during the day and follow my nutrition plan perfectly. To all appearances, I seemed to have finally gotten control of my eating habits. But I had a secret. Late at night, when my daughters were asleep and my husband was working out of town, I would chew and spit out whole pies, bags of hamburgers and french fries, ice cream, candy bars—you name it. I would chew them to the point of swallowing and spit everything out into zip lock freezer bags. Then I would seal them and hide them outside in the bottom of the trash can. I would do this sometimes for hours at a time, until I was exhausted and my jaws would ache. I had the body I wanted, but my spiritual life and my emotions were a wreck. I had tremendous guilt about this eating addiction, but I couldn't seem to stop. I hated my compulsions and addictions. I hated myself.

Before I could truly change and begin to like myself again, I had to change my thinking. I had to let go of thinking that I had to be perfect to be somebody worthwhile. I had to focus on Jesus so He could make me complete in Him. I had to begin seeking His kingdom first so that He was the most important thing in my life.

As I began to focus on my Heavenly Father, I found comfort. And as I delved into His Word, I found strength, freedom and healing. What I learned is that there has to be balance between your spirit, soul and body. God wants all three to be well. In Romans 12:1, Paul says, "I beseech you therefore, brethren, by the mercies of God, that you present your bodies a living sacrifice, holy, acceptable to God, which is your *reasonable* service" (NKJV).

Before, I had tried every unreasonable thing promoted on late night television to keep my weight in check. Now, I trust the Father to speak truth to me and lead me into reasonable service. Reasonable service creates balance. Reasonable service creates peace. Romans 8:11 says, "But if the Spirit of Him who raised Jesus from the dead dwells in you, He who raised Christ from the dead will also give life to your mortal bodies through His Spirit who dwells in you" (NKJV).

That is where the power comes from to defeat addictions. Christian friends, the power that raised Jesus from the dead is inside of you!

Because I have given my body to God, He is in charge of it. It is no longer reasonable for me to obsess over my weight. It is no longer reasonable to work on food preparation and exercise for three hours a day and give God the leftover five minutes before I fall asleep. At the same time, it is no longer reasonable that I sit on the couch all day because I'm so overweight I don't have any extra energy to serve God working for His kingdom. It's no longer reasonable that I'm so focused on myself and my appearance that I don't see the needs of others.

I'm happy to say that now when Satan brings temptations to practice old behaviors, I know the power that God has given me and I can send the enemy packing! I have found freedom in exercising moderation and there is so much more peace in my life.

Because I know what it's like to be fat and sick, and have learned how great it feels to be strong and healthy, I have an intense passion to assist others in their journey towards optimal health. I am excited that I am able to show people how to live a balanced life. By being sensitive to the Holy Spirit's leading, I am able to develop a plan for a weight loss that will work for each individual. And as was prophesied over me many years ago, I've been privileged to lay hands on individuals and see them healed.

I'm not a spectacular person because I lost 90 pounds. I just started putting one foot in front of the other and started walking toward my TRUE healing. I still have to walk it out every single day. It wasn't just the physical weight that was holding me back—I needed a spiritual healing and I needed Jesus to heal my broken emotions.

In February 2012, I developed the 4-week *Losing IT* sermon series with my pastor to encourage my church family to get healthy, both physically and spiritually. The Fit for Freedom Challenge which followed was a way to share the insights that God had given me with those who felt they were ready for a longer, more intensive program.

Many lives were changed during the challenge. I am including some of those stories, along with testimonies from some former NBC's *The Biggest Loser* and ABC's *Extreme Weight Loss* contestants I've worked with on various projects to encourage you on your own fitness journey. My prayer is that as you read about what God has done for them and continues to do in them, you will be inspired to make positive changes in your own life.

As you start this book, would you ask Jesus to help you drop more than just the excess pounds? Ask Him to help you let go of the things that are holding you back from doing what you have been gifted to do. Then you'll begin to discover your true calling and God-given purpose in life. I did—and I know you can, too!

DAY 1

Get in Over Your Head

They saw the works of the LORD,
his wonderful deeds in the deep.

Psalms 107:24

I can't tell you how excited I am that you have decided to take this journey with God over the next 30 days! As you begin this devotional, I want to encourage you not to play it safe! Stand up in the face of fear, failure, your past, "the way it used to be," soreness and pain, and wade right out into the deep water. Keep going until you are in over head and don't look back. Dog paddle if you have to, it's okay. Soon you will be swimming with confidence!

Physical fitness prepares us to take on life's pressures and prepares us mentally and spiritually to fight Satan's attacks. I will be your guide on your journey to good health, but the Holy Spirit will play the ultimate role of Helper, Teacher, and Convictor. Listen to Him.

I can teach you everything I know and I can push you, but if the Holy Spirit isn't involved, this will be just a nice little book you picked up and read this month. My vision for you is that the time you invest in worshiping God with your body through exercise and good nutrition will impact you so greatly that you will see the positive effects of it in your marriage, in your temperament, in your service to God, in your personal relationship with Him, in your energy level, and in a greater desire to reach out and share Christ with others. I know it can happen because it happened to me!

The Bible says that our bodies are the temple of the Holy Spirit. Expect to see the wonders of God when you have been obedient to get your Temple in order. I believe it is no accident that you have chosen this particular time to work on getting healthy. God has put us together for a purpose. He knows exactly what you are capable of and His timing is perfect!

> *Heavenly Father, thank you for Your Word that shows the way to good health. Holy Spirit, I rest in You. Guide me as I work to become physically fit.*

IN IT FOR THE LONG HAUL

My daughter and I made it to The Biggest Loser finals. We were so excited and had all of our friends and family praying for us and cheering us on through the entire process. When we left for California, we had all of our affairs in order for the next six months. Alexandra had taken the semester off from college because we were sure we were going all the way. I was unemployed at the time so the timing was perfect.

When they knocked on our hotel door, I'm not sure why, but I knew they were sending us home. Devastated cannot even begin to explain how we felt. For the next week, I could barely get out of bed. I had so many hopes and dreams wrapped up in making it on the show and now I was back home, still fat, unemployed, rejected and feeling like I had let my daughter down. For the next few months, depression was my best friend. I didn't want to leave my house, I didn't want to see my friends, and I certainly didn't care what I ate.

Then in January, my friend Kathleen said she saw an ad in a magazine that they were going to be having some of *The Biggest Loser* contestants at a local church and asked if I want to go. Did I? I wasn't sure. I wanted to meet them; but I wanted to *be* them, too. I ended up going all four weeks of the series because I knew I needed to do something—anything. After seeing all the former contestants, I knew that I had to get moving. I was getting to a weight where I could barely move. Everything was uncomfortable. My stomach hit the steering wheel of my car. I could barely walk up a flight a stairs, and forget about exercising. I could maybe make it two houses down and I felt like I had asthma!

So, I was determined to do this when I joined Laurie's program. The first week, I did what was suggested and drank nothing but water. Ninety days later, 99% of what I drink is plain old water. Thanks to the goal setting, for the past three weeks I have been walking three times a week and I feel better than ever. I have counted every single morsel of food that has passed my lips over the past 90 days and this morning I finally weighed myself...27 pounds...gone forever. And in the next 90 days, I will shed 27 more. I can do this!

I am now gainfully employed, feeling 100% better than I was 5 months ago, physically, emotionally and spiritually. Through Laurie's teaching, I have come to trust that God has my back (even when I question why

He does some things). He had a different journey for me than the one I thought, but it has been a fantastic one.

Laurie Graves and all the others who have volunteered their time will never really know how grateful I am and how you all helped kick start me on the fit girl path. I have a ways to go…but man, do I have momentum!

Thank you!

Margret Mowery

Update: Margret has now lost over 100 pounds, has a wonderful job and is inspiring others in her family and workplace to get fit!

DAY 2

The Right Start

What agreement is there between the
temple of God and idols? For we are the
temple of the living God.
As God has said:
"I will live with them
and walk among them,
and I will be their God,
and they will be my people."

2 Corinthians 6:16

Day Two of your journey to good health, and I can hear you complaining already. "Come on, already. Give us the list! Show us the food we're supposed to eat, tell us what exercises to do, give us the steps so we can bust 30 pounds off in 30 days!" Okay, I'm going to. Here you go, step one…

Start with communion. Probably didn't see that one coming, did you? Were you even aware that you could take communion all by yourself? You can, and you should, as you start this devotional. Be moved to repentance for not caring for your body in a way that is pleasing to God. Once you have repented for your disobedience, you may have some emotional baggage to deal with.

Eating issues are part of a package that includes emotional wounds and addictive behaviors. If you have been dealing with these problems for a long time, you are going to have to start engaging in spiritual warfare to get that stronghold out of your life. Spiritual warfare includes prayer, fasting, and reading God's Word.

The Bible says that once you become a Christian, the Holy Spirit comes and dwells inside of you. Your body becomes His temple. Second Corinthians 6:16 says that since you are the temple of the living God, there can be no agreement between your body and idols. Anything that is preventing you from having a strong, healthy body must be vanquished. If food is your idol, that idol must be torn down. If television is your idol, it must be destroyed. (Don't smash your 55" flatscreen. I'm speaking figuratively.) Whatever is coming between you and God's will for your life must be submitted to Him.

Take some time today to submit your will and your desires to the Father. As Paul exhorted the church at Rome, "Therefore, I urge you, brothers and sisters, in view of God's mercy, to offer your bodies as a living sacrifice, holy and pleasing to God—this is your true and proper worship" (Romans 12:1).

> *Heavenly Father, I give my life to You. I give You my brokenness, my addiction, my pain, my cravings, my hopes, my dreams—I give it all to You, Lord. Take the pieces of my life and put me back together stronger, better and happier than before as I obey Your will and build this temple.*

BEING CONSECRATED KEEPS HER ON THE RIGHT PATH

Three years ago, my husband Steve and I purchased a garden center. It was a bit of a dream come true for Steve who had always wanted to have his own business. I wasn't all that thrilled because it is 85 miles away from our home. Obviously, Steve has to be hands-on at the garden center and it is too far for a daily commute. So Steve lives away and comes home two days out of the week, usually a Thursday and a Sunday. I continue to teach school and take care of our son, Travis, who is in high school.

To make a long story short, I became very bored, depressed and lonely. I have been reasonably active throughout my life, but as I got older things hurt, so I didn't work out very much. This became a cycle of being too tired to do anything about being tired! My thoughts became very dark.

When I heard about the fitness program, I knew I had to participate. Through the Fit for Freedom Challenge I have gotten my butt off the couch and kept my hands out of the chip bag. I also spend considerably more time in God's Word. It really opened my eyes to see the sin and lies in my life that I had used as excuses for inactivity and laziness, both physically and spiritually.

Thank you for this challenge. I know each session is a true labor of love and you're an inspiration to me.

I also wanted to tell you that the first session really laid the foundation for me. You talked about "first things first" and we took the Lord's Supper together. Whenever I felt like giving up, I remembered that we had consecrated ourselves and this journey to the Lord and that kept me moving forward.

Thanks again,
Shirley Gent
P.S. I also lost 15 pounds!

DAY 3

Get Ready to Fight

The weapons we fight with are not the weapons of the world. On the contrary, they have divine power to demolish strongholds. We demolish arguments and every pretension that sets itself up against the knowledge of God, and we take captive every thought to make it obedient to Christ.

2 Corinthians 10:4-5

There is a battlefield in your mind. Every day the enemy will come and try to tell you:

- how pitiful you are
- how unlovable you are
- how fat you are
- how you'll never be free
- how you'll never amount to anything, etc.

Satan sometimes puts lies like these in your mind and sometimes he has another person speak them into your life. In that moment, you have a decision—you can dwell on that thought or you can combat it with God's word. If Satan can get you to dwell on the lie long enough, it will drop into your heart. Then you begin believing the lie and it becomes truth to you. You start speaking that lie with your mouth. Matthew 12:34 says, "The mouth speaks what the heart is full of." What has your mouth been speaking? Have you been saying negative things about yourself?

What you play over and over in your mind and say out of your mouth will significantly impact your ability to have freedom from strongholds. You have a choice to cast enemy thoughts away. You can "take every thought captive" and make them line up with what God says about you—that you are "fearfully and wonderfully made" (Psalms 139:14).

I want to warn you that the enemy does not want you healthy. He does not want your emotional wounds to be healed. He will fight really hard to keep you sick and stupid. Because Satan knows that once you are free from your inner pain, crippling addictions and excess weight, you could be dangerous. You could get off the couch and start doing exceptional things for God.

Of course, you would have to let go of some things first. We are a wounded people. Many have been wounded by a parent, a spouse or another person we trusted. The enemy loves to use these wounds to keep us bound. He wants us to be tied to the past, always looking back and never moving forward. There comes a time when you have to decide. Are you going to continue rolling in the pain and the mess? Or are you going to get up, let Jesus dust you off, and let Him heal your wounds so that you can start a new life of freedom?

What will it be? I pray that you decide to let Jesus help you regain your life—spirit, soul and body.

> *Lord Jesus, thank you for taking all my sin and shame on the cross. I give my life to You. Help me to live a life that is pleasing to You.*

TRANSFORMED TO LIVE: BIGGEST LOSER CONTESTANT, KEN ANDREWS

LIFE. DEATH. Have you ever noticed that when we face death, it puts life into perspective? In 2008, I almost died of sepsis. It was an experience that shook me and started me on a journey to find help. Through some very fortunate circumstances, my son Austin and I were chosen for season 11 of NBC's The Biggest Loser show. I had arrived at the show at 377 lbs., on 11 medications and trying to survive day-to-day. I was not really living. I was merely existing.

A few weeks into the show, on one of our daily hikes in the hills of Malibu, I experienced the beginning of my transformation—a transformation that began with an encounter with God. Thumbing through my iPod Shuffle, I flipped to an unfamiliar song and heard these words:

> *It's time for healing, time to move on*
> *It's time to fix what's been broken too long*
> *Time to make right what has been wrong*
> *It's time to find my way to where I belong*
> *There's a wave that's crashing over me*
> *And all I can do is surrender*

> *Whatever You're doing inside of me*
> *It feels like chaos but somehow there's peace*
> *It's hard to surrender to what I can't see*
> *But I'm giving in to something Heavenly.*

By this time, the tears had begun to flow. I knew that I had encountered God, and that this moment was a divine appointment. The music continued:

> *Time for a milestone*
> *Time to begin again*
> *Reevaluate who I really am*
> *Am I doing everything to follow Your will*
> *Or just climbing aimlessly over these hills?*[1]

And there, on the hills of Malibu, I was on my knees in the dirt. Sobbing. Wailing. The dam had broken and the tears flowed. I had encountered God and He loved me. Physically broken down, emotionally struggling me. From that day on, I started each day with a hike or a walk, met God, and continued weeping from around the middle of October through the end of January.

But transformation is hard. Losing the weight required exercise, eating only the right things, and rest. Day after day, week after week.

Even more than the hard physical work, the emotional healing and inner transformation process was extremely taxing. Weeping, toiling, writing, remembering clearly through the tears and pain—it was at times agonizingly difficult, but essential for this journey. I meditated on particular scriptures that allowed me to deeply understand them, and to make them not only promises from God's Word, but real promises from God to me. I had been running from my past but finally had stopped running and had turned to face it with God's help.

Though the process was long and hard, I began to see changes. The tears that had started as tears of repentance and regret became tears of gratitude. I had faced my past and had come to grips with it. God had changed my life from the inside out. The Ken Andrews who left home to go on the *Biggest Loser* show was not the same Ken Andrews who returned home.

I had finally really come to God—brokenness and all. I had been so weary, so burdened. I let go of the need to try to fix everyone's problems and carry all their burdens for them; I was coming out the other end of this journey a changed person.

I ask you—what obstacle or issue in your life hinders you most? What would your life look like a year from now if you overcame that obstacle or issue? This can happen. I'm living proof of it. Two years ago I would have told you that the best years of my life were behind me. I now know that is not true.

The best years of your life can be ahead of you, too. Your journey will be different, but you will find the same God, the same restoration and the same freedom I have found. Yes, I lost weight, but my weight loss was simply the by-product of emotional, spiritual and physical health.

This devotional is an excellent tool that can help you find that place of balance; the place where you are truly whole in every facet of life including your physical body. Just stick with it!

Ken Andrews
Founder of RetroFit Ministries
Former Contestant on NBC's
The Biggest Loser, Season 11

---

[1] Sanctus Real. "Whatever You're Doing (Something Real)." *We Need Each Other*. Sparrow/EMD, 2008.

DAY 4

Transformation Begins with Self-Respect

Do you not know that your bodies are temples of the Holy Spirit, who is in you, whom you have received from God? You are not your own; you were bought at a price. Therefore honor God with your bodies.

1 Corinthians 6:19-20

Joan Didion once said, "Self-respect is a question of recognizing that anything worth having has a price." Whenever you start a journey of change there can be great opposition. It can come in many different forms—family criticism, sabotaging friends, and blatant attacks of the enemy. Anything that is worth having is going to have a cost associated with it.

Many women I know will not obey their Heavenly Father concerning their weight and health because it will cause a rift with their husband who is a "meat and potatoes" kind of a guy. I'm not suggesting that you should put your diet ahead of your husband. But I don't believe in excuses either. There are many creative ways to make comfort food healthy.

Opposition can come from other fronts, too. You may have friends who will belittle you when you begin your new eating plan. Co-workers may seem to purposely have more lunch celebrations now that one of their own is fighting the battle of the bulge. And, of course, Satan will try to push you off the path with thoughts of failure and discouragement before you even get started. The secret is to have enough self-respect that you disregard these negative comments.

Here are a few keys to help you receive your transformation and gain self-respect:

1. Stay true to where you feel the Holy Spirit is leading you as you start your nutrition and fitness program.
2. Pick a support team of two or three people whom you know will encourage and pray for you. Let them know some specific ways to help.
3. Write out some scriptures on index cards and have them in your wallet or purse to pull out and meditate on when adversity strikes.
4. Have some key verses memorized to replace the negative thoughts Satan brings.
5. Plan your meals. If you have a plan you are less likely to be tempted to ignore the strategy the Holy Spirit has given you.
6. Plan your exercise on a calendar. You'll be less likely to blow it off if you manage it as an appointment.

Transformation is a daily process. It involves laying down your flesh to achieve God's best for your life. It may not feel good at the time, but the self-respect that comes from pushing through and accomplishing your goals is priceless!

Heavenly Father, I want to honor You with my body. I want to have a beautiful, sturdy temple for the Holy Spirit. Give me the courage and conviction I need each day to be obedient to Your will.

SPIRITUALLY FIT

I wanted to make sure you know what a blessing your program has been for me! I have made positive changes in my diet and physical activity that are already new habits. And while that is exciting and I feel awesome, the even better part is the change I have made in my spiritual walk, too.

I am more consistently seeking God's direction and guidance in my decisions and my thoughts. It is so special and freeing! I also have an amazing witness as I share what I have learned. There are several people in my office making healthy changes, too, so God is giving me divine appointments almost every day.

Praise to our awesome God for inspiring this program and for His ever-present power that enabled my life-changing experience! I had my quarterly diabetes check up today and A1C was down from 7.6 in Feb to 6.9! That is the lowest I have ever had! And my doctor's words for my cholesterol: "Awesome! Keep up whatever you are doing!" The Fit for Freedom Challenge has been a huge blessing to me.

Becky French

Update: Becky and her family prepare healthy meals and all go to the gym together. She no longer needs cholesterol medicine, takes less insulin and recently completed her first ever 5K race!

DAY 5

Go Ahead and Eat!

Then a voice told him, "Get up, Peter.
Kill and eat."
"Surely not, Lord!" Peter replied. "I have never eaten
anything impure or unclean."
The voice spoke to him a second time, "Do not call
anything impure that God has made clean."

Acts 10:13–15

Cornelius, a captain of the Italian army, sent his servants to invite the apostle Peter to stay at his house. Before the servants arrived, Peter was praying and fell into a trance. He saw a huge sheet dropping from the sky filled with all kinds of animals. God told Peter to eat them, but Peter was confused and said, "No, Lord, they aren't kosher. I can't eat unclean food." God's voice came again and said to Peter, "If *I* say it's okay, it's okay."

While Peter was still pondering the meaning of his vision, the servants arrived to deliver Cornelius' invitation. Since the Italian captain was a gentile, he was considered unclean by the Jews and devout Jews like Peter would not normally associate with him.

Many people interpret the trance as God telling Peter that he should go to Cornelius' house because all believers are equal. I believe that is true. But here is how the Holy Spirit had me start looking at this passage: I believe

God superseded the Jewish law so that Peter could have freedom in fellowship with Cornelius and not offend his host.

Have you ever invited someone to dinner who was on a low-carb diet and they picked all of the noodles out of your lasagna or casserole like they were radioactive? It's offensive, right?

Here's what I want you to see...

Cornelius asked Peter to stay for a few days and he didn't have to worry about whether the food was clean or unclean. Peter had not traveled with his kosher food divided into Tupperware. He didn't bring baggies of unleavened bread. He was not freaking out because he forgot his supplements or didn't have his filtered water.

God had shown Peter in a vision that He was going to bless him physically and spiritually no matter what he ate. That is freedom, my friends—doing your part so God can do His. You can trust the Father with your health and your food choices!

> *Thank you, Heavenly Father, for caring more about people than about rules. Help me to live each day in a way that shows Your love to other people.*

A TYRANT NO LONGER

As a personal trainer, I was excited when I started helping Laurie with her program at our church because I would be able to help those who were struggling with their weight. After the first night I realized that it was going to be so much more than that. I discovered very quickly that I was having just as many issues with balance in my life as many of them were. I was on the other end of the spectrum though.

No matter how well I ate I still felt it wasn't good enough. I still felt overweight even though I had 7% body fat. I couldn't enjoy fellowship over a meal with family and friends any longer because I was judging those I was eating with. I was constantly thinking, "How can they be eating that?" I was becoming a tyrant about nutrition with my wife and kids.

Because of Laurie's teaching, I learned to start letting go and trusting the Lord with my food. I still eat well, but I'm learning to have more balance with my passion for fitness and nutrition. I'm getting better about letting others make their own decisions in my family. It's not easy because I love them so much I want them to be super healthy. But I'm learning to turn it over to the Lord and love them unconditionally.

The other thing that was new to me was walking for exercise. I'd never done low-intensity cardio before. I started leading a walking group two nights a week and fell in love with the simplicity of walking. It was a getaway for my mind and spirit and I continued it on my own as a quiet time with the Lord. I saw so many people receive spiritual healing and lose lifelong burdens through the Fit for Freedom program. I am honored to have been a part of it and very grateful for all those who participated with me and accepted me for me.

Chad Griffin

DAY 6

See Your Success

*In the desert the whole community
grumbled against Moses and Aaron. The Israelites
said to them, "If only we had died by the LORD's
hand in Egypt! There we sat around pots of meat
and ate all the food we wanted, but you have
brought us out into this desert to starve this entire
assembly to death."*

Exodus 16:2–3

About a month and a half after God delivered the children of Israel out of slavery in Egypt, they began to tire of short rations. They complained to Moses, "Why didn't God allow us to die in Egypt where we had lamb stew and all the bread we could eat?"

It is interesting that nothing has changed over the centuries. Forty-five days is the average length of time that a person stays on a diet. We can usually say "no" to our flesh for about six weeks, and then we are done. We begin looking back to our former way of eating and longing for some of the good old bad stuff.

When you are on a diet, do you keep looking back at McDonald's or Wendy's like the Israelites looked back to the land of Egypt and longed for their combo meals? Do you yearn to eat a whole gallon of ice cream? Do you wish you could still supersize your fries?

The Israelites wandered for 40 years in the desert because they refused to follow God. Some of you have wandered for years trying to find a new way to get rid of an addiction. Let me share a time-tested secret to success: keep your eyes forward, stop looking back, and allow God to lead you to your deliverance.

The only way to be successful in eating for better health is to quit turning around and looking back at your Egypt. Instead, get a vision of the new place God wants to take you—your Promised Land. See yourself as thin and healthy, and keep that picture foremost in your thoughts. Remain focused on the dream that God has placed in your heart, keep looking ahead and allow the power of God to guide you. You will reach your goal sooner than you ever imagined.

> *Lord, you are my Provider. I trust You to give me what I need. Holy Spirit, please help me to control the desires of my flesh so that my body can become a strong, healthy temple that is pleasing to You.*

NEW BODY, NEW LIFE

First and foremost, I want to give all the glory and praise to God for bringing me thus far. I know that I could not have achieved what I have done without Him. As Philippians 4:13 says, "I know that I can do all things because of the strength He gives."

When I began my journey, I weighed in at 323 lbs. It seems like a lot now that I look back. But in just a few months, I am now at 274 lbs! If you would have asked me at the beginning of the year if I would be where I am now, I would have laughed and said, "I wish!" But God is an amazing God! Little did I know that Laurie would plant the seed which I believe made it possible for ME!

It started with the *Losing IT* sermon series, and seeing members of our congregation take a leap of faith and put their weight out there for all to see during weekly weigh-ins on stage. The most inspirational contestant to me was Jodi. I felt closest to her, because I, too, was over 300 lbs. After that first sermon, I knew I had to do something! And then the offer for the Fit for Freedom Challenge was made. I was excited, and I believed that God was speaking to me to join. I knew it was my time, even though up to the last minute of the kick-off meeting I was making excuses. In the end, God won and I showed up. It was a day that changed my life!

The first meeting was so inspirational. I knew after that first meeting that I was on the right track to healing. Not just with my weight issues, but in mind, body and spirit. Throughout the meetings, getting to hear teaching on how to care for my body as the temple of the Holy Spirit continually made my life take on new meaning. The peace and happiness I now feel, feeling better both inside and out...well, there are just NO words.

My health has drastically changed. My doctor was surprised at how much my blood sugar had improved. A year ago, my A1c was 8.5. Two weeks after starting the challenge, it was 6.1! The doctor took me off half of one of my medicine dosage and completely off one of my other diabetic medications. Every time I check my sugar levels, they are better. Getting off the anti-depressant was a big step, too. Looking back, I can't even imagine that I needed it!

This is just the beginning of my journey. I have a goal and I know that this time I will see it through. During the challenge, I found solace in prayer, friendships and accountability. Thank you from the bottom of my heart.

Melissa Norman

Melissa lost 49.5 pounds and 41.5 inches in 12 weeks and was the grand prize winner of the challenge. Through her weight loss she's found confidence to start college and pursue a degree in Criminal Justice!

DAY 7

Fast for Better Health

"Please test your servants for ten days:
Give us nothing but vegetables to eat and water to
drink. Then compare our appearance with that of the
young men who eat the royal food, and treat your
servants in accordance with what you see." So he
agreed to this and tested them for ten days.
At the end of the ten days they looked healthier and
better nourished than any of the young men who ate
the royal food.

Daniel 1:12-15

Daniel determined that he would not defile himself with the king's meat that had been sacrificed to idols. His three Jewish friends decided to do the same.

They agreed to fast meat altogether and eat nothing but vegetables and drink only water for ten days straight. Fortunately, Daniel was able to persuade the kitchen steward to help them remain true to their commitment to God.

At the end of ten days, the four were inspected and were proven to be superior to all of the other young men. The king himself tested them and found them to be stronger and ten times smarter than all of his wise men.

Soon, the king had a crazy dream that kept him awake all night. Only Daniel was able to interpret the meaning of the dream. He had removed the distraction of his stomach and gained something greater—strength and wisdom.

Sometimes you may feel as if your brain cells aren't all firing. You have "brain fog," forgetfulness, sleeplessness, and other problems. Much of that could be due to the enormous amounts of preservatives, sugar and artificial products that you have consumed over the years. Cleaning up the foods that you place in your mouth can help heal you mentally, physically, and spiritually.

Fasting has become a regular part of my life. Sometimes I fast certain foods, and sometimes it's a meal or several meals, but I have seen God move in very powerful ways in my life since I started fasting.

God has broken some major strongholds for me and grown my spiritual life as a result of setting aside food in order to hear from Him. What could God do in your life if you said "no" to your stomach for His glory?

> *Lord, I love You more than I love food. I want to hear from You more than I want anything else. Speak to me when I fast and pray, seeking Your will and Your direction for my life. I will obey Your leading.*

FLYER LEADS TO FITNESS AND FAITH

My family stumbled upon Laurie Graves and Northwood Church by coming across a flyer in the mail that advertised the upcoming *Losing IT* series, featuring some Biggest Loser contestants. We were looking for a new church and also at a place in life where we wanted and needed to get healthy, so this was a perfect opportunity. What happened in the following weeks has literally changed my family's lives as well as impacted the lives of our friends.

My mother and I decided to join the fitness program to lose weight and we invited some of our friends to join the class with us. During those 12 weeks, I realized that my life and health are extremely important. I learned tons of information from Laurie and the other trainers and became part of a community of people that were serious about getting their physical lives in order. For the first time in my life, I started exercising consistently and actually looked forward to it! I began cooking more and actually enjoyed that as well! New friendships were formed and existing ones were strengthened and my relationship with God became a priority in my life again. I loved that during the Fit for Freedom Challenge Laurie provided a perfect mix of Bible teaching, nutritional information, exercise tips, accountability time, and "heart" work. Instead of just hearing instruction and leaving class not knowing what my next steps were, I was taught by her how to take everything I was learning and put it into practice in my daily life. And I began to see results.

As a result of the fitness challenge, I lost 20 lbs and numerous inches. I laid aside my daily addiction to soda and saw a drastic improvement with my migraines and daily headaches. I gained confidence in myself and my abilities. I discovered that I have an interest in learning about food and how to eat "clean." I was inspired to begin teaching my 3-year-old healthy eating habits starting right now, in hopes that she will not have the same struggles with weight and food that I do. Overall, I felt very good about myself and my life during that time and was so happy that I had found someone to look up to regarding this difficult life-long battle.

During the last few months, I have began to struggle again and gain a little of my weight back. However, I have not and will not give up. I look at this time as just a season that will soon pass. I will never go back to the woman I was before the challenge. That is not an option. I have continued taking multiple fitness/Bible study classes with Laurie and they serve as a lifeline to me. Her gentle spirit and authenticity continually inspires me to be a better person. Every time I am around her, this motivation rises up in me to take charge of my life and health and to go out and live my dreams.

Whether it is through exercise classes, bible studies or nutritional classes, I plan to be a student of Laurie's until it is my time to become a teacher. She is an amazing woman of God and I am truly blessed to have her in my life. I am so thankful that God placed that flyer in our mail and the desire in our hearts to follow His lead. Our lives have been impacted forever due to that event!

Carey Casey

DAY 8

Be a Superhero

*My brethren, if any among you strays from
the truth and one turns him back, let him know that
he who turns a sinner from the error of his way will
save his soul from death and will
cover a multitude of sins.*

James 5:19–20

Lot, Abraham's nephew, lived in Sodom. God warned him that it was time to leave that sinful city, but he was used to the sin. In fact, he participated in the wickedness even though he knew better. At one point in the story, the city was burning down all around him and he still didn't want to leave! An angel had to come and take his hand and actually pull him from the city. God cared enough about Lot to snatch him out of the destruction even though Lot wasn't eager to be saved.

A friend of mine who is a medic told me that he was recently called to go out with a team to remove a 1,100-pound man from his home and transport him to the hospital because he was having an irregular heartbeat. Eight men were required to transport him. After examining him, the doctors told him he had only days to live.

At the hospital, the morbidly obese patient's weight exceeded the capacity of even the largest bariatric hospital bed. The poor man was terribly ashamed of his size.

He cried and begged the medics to take him back to his home, because he didn't want to die in humiliation. The ambulance team took pity on him and transported him back to his home where he died within 30 minutes. He was only 30 years old.

I can't help but wonder what life could have been like for this young man if someone had been willing to snatch him from his destruction. What if he had had someone in his life who cared enough to give him a helping hand? What if his family had said, "No, we will not bring you unhealthy food for you to eat in bed because we love you too much to let you eat yourself to death?" What if someone had been willing to see that he got professional help?

As you continue on your journey to better physical and spiritual health, God will use the things you learn in order to help someone. Count on it. Look for the opportunity, because it's going to happen. You just have to be willing to reach out and lend a hand to a hurting individual. Sometimes that person may not even realize that they need to be rescued, but as you share your own story, it may be the catalyst they need to make lasting positive change—change that might even save their life.

> *Lord, open my eyes to the pain of those around me. Show me how I can demonstrate your love to a hurting soul. Use me, Father, to make a difference for your kingdom.*

TAKING THE FIRST STEP

Starting this journey was the hardest part. Jeremy, my son, has lost 90 pounds. I'll never forget the day I asked him why he had lost the weight he did. He reminded me of a funeral of a friend we had attended. The father passed away and his kids who were my son's age no longer had their dad. Jeremy said he wanted me around for a long time. He told me that he had lost his weight hoping it would encourage me to do the same.

When the *Losing IT* series started I just kept hearing, "I want you around, Dad." At Northwood Church, we had two teams who competed to lose weight for the series and I was picked for one of the teams. My starting weight was 275 pounds, the most I have ever weighed.

I want to share with you what made this possible for me other than working out and changing my eating habits. First, it is so important to have people support what you are trying to do. My family was crucial to my weight loss. My kids encouraged me and my wife Anna changed the meals we ate (and made them taste amazing!). My small group at church constantly encouraged me. When I said I was struggling with a workout, they would tell me things like, "You can do it, Rudy—it's only 14 songs on your iPod." They did whatever they could to keep me motivated.

The last thing that I want to mention is how the Father walked with me through this. During the hour-long workouts I prayed, worshiped and listened to amazing messages of His goodness. The one that stands out the most is the first thing the Father told me when I started the program and was praying about it early in the process. He led me to this scripture and told me clearly, without a doubt, He would do this for me. Ephesians 3:20: "Now to him who is able to do immeasurably more than all we ask or imagine, according to his power that is at work within us, be the glory."

It took me 48 years to gain the weight and I knew it would take a lot of work to get it off. But the Father said, "I can heal the sick, make the blind to see. Straighten out a wayward father or mother. I can help you be healthy again, physically, mentally and spiritually." The Heavenly Father did that for me. He'll do it for you. Just do the hardest part...get started...NOW!

Rudy Carrasco

Update: Rudy has now lost a total of 60 pounds and is feeling more energetic than he has in years!

DAY 9

Freedom from Negative Thinking

*It is for freedom that Christ has set us free. Stand
firm, then, and do not let yourselves be burdened
again by a yoke of slavery.*

Galatians 5:1

I stand on this scripture every day. In the past, I had
trained myself to be so disciplined that I was walking in
bondage and neglecting fellowship with others. I was tormented when I gained a pound. I would stand in front of
the mirror and ridicule God's creation. I was in total slavery. I had accepted Christ, but I chose to remain in the
same yoke and chains that the enemy had captured and
secured me in. I continued to have the kind of negative
thoughts had that started forming at the age of ten when
one of my "friends" told me I was fat and nobody would
ever marry me.

How did God help me transform that pattern of
thinking? I had to actively create new thought patterns. I
had to meditate on God's thoughts concerning me. I had
to read scripture. I had to seek out friends who would
encourage me, and I had to stop thinking and speaking
negative thoughts over myself. It's a process and a healing
that I'm still walking out today. With God's help, I take

hold of the thoughts the enemy brings as soon as I recognize them and cast them down. 2 Corinthians 10:5 is an excellent verse that illustrates this process: "We demolish arguments and every pretension that sets itself up against the knowledge of God, and we take captive every thought to make it obedient to Christ."

Be encouraged that there is freedom for you. There is no need to stay enslaved to Satan anymore!

Read this confession out loud over yourself today:

> *I am wonderfully made by God! I cast down every thought and imagination that tries to exalt itself over the knowledge of Christ that says I am made in His image and that I am beautifully and wonderfully made. I will fill my spirit and mind with scripture to combat the enemy's attacks in my thought life. I will resist him, knowing that all the enemy can do is lie because he is the father of all lies. He NEVER brings truth to me. Today I build myself up in faith by speaking words of truth over myself: "I am amazing." "I am unique." "I am powerful in Christ and I have a gift that God can only deliver through me." In Jesus's name, amen.*

SOMETHING BIG

The truth is I struggle with my weight. I always have. I have had weight issues since I was a freshman in high school. I am an adopted child. I was placed in foster care at the age of 18 months and I was adopted into a family at the age of four. These alone could have been factors in weight gain, but on top of that I was severely physically and emotionally abused. The beatings and the demeaning words planted a spirit of underachievement in my soul. I wanted to do great things with my life, but I set myself up for failure and lacked sufficient confidence to become who God made me to be. Through a series of hurtful interactions with friends and family I began to gain weight and had ballooned up to 350 pounds by my junior year of high school. I absolutely loved choir and I loved being in the school musicals, but I lacked the confidence to shine.

Fast forward to college and here is the perfect picture of a boy who so desperately wanted to excel and be accepted for who he was, but was held back by his lack of confidence. I found love, and got married to the most wonderfully beautiful girl the world has ever seen. She is the most non-judgmental, caring, compassionate, authentic, loving, beautiful person I have ever known. We have a beautiful son, Greysen, and two daughters, Ella and Jillian. I was happier than ever before, but the weight wasn't coming off because I wasn't addressing the problem. In fact, I had done a good job of sweeping it all under the rug. In May of 2009, I weighed in at 444 pounds. I was a Type 2 Diabetic and didn't know it. I was killing myself and I had no idea I was doing it.

That year, 2009, I lost 155 pounds during the taping and airing of *The Biggest Loser* season 8. It was a huge year for me. I felt confident, sure and ready to tackle life. In 2010, I went on to lose another 40 pounds, bringing my total weight loss to a staggering 205 pounds! It was an exciting time in my life and I felt like NOTHING could stop my momentum and break my stride. I was wrong.

I have been a full time pastor since 2007. Everything seemed to be going well and then the tidal wave of adversity crashed in. The person I worked for at the church became a very strong adversary. For some reason, things changed and I was no longer needed, or even more hurtful, wanted at the church. I had been on cloud nine just months before—finishing half-marathons, marathons, and heading up the Health and Wellness ministry at the church, then BAM! A wall. I wasn't sure what God was doing, but from January of 2011 until August 2011 I endured some of the most stressful times in my life. I felt worthless and I turned back to the old friend that had always helped me through the hard times—food. Food that could make my belly feel full and comforted. I ate. I didn't go to gym. I didn't run outside. I wasn't allowed to travel and speak anymore because of the job criteria that changed, so I hid. I was able to hide and numb out and not do a thing.

Fast forward to the *Losing IT* series at Northwood. I had contracted with Laurie Graves and Northwood Church to come speak at this event a year before. I felt like I had an obligation to fulfill the promise I made to her to come and speak. I did, and even at a weight gain of 60 lbs, she was kind, compassionate and loving. I had so expected judgmental looks from the audience, and it was driving me crazy. That is the opposite of what happened. The church was a warm, receptive place of grace and love. I realized that weekend that God had me on a path of strength and conditioning. Not the kind of physical strength and conditioning I was used to, but emotional strength and conditioning.

Through this experience and a counseling program a few months earlier where I regained my confidence and got in touch with my heart, I learned that I am a fun, loving, compassionate child of God. That's it. Nothing more, nothing less. I'm not a number on a scale. I'm not a television show contestant. I'm not a gauge. I'm not a guru. I'm not a know-it-all weight loss expert, I'm not a celebrity. I'm not better than anyone else. I am an overcomer. I am a child of God who is redeemed. I am a beautiful part of God's poetry that's sung over me while I sleep at night. I am a husband and father who wants to be better at both. I am a brother, I am a friend. But most importantly, I am God's child, loved and held each second, each hour of each beautiful day.

The Northwood *Losing IT* program was a catalyst for a renewed spirit, soul, body and mind. Recently I did something that was on my bucket list. I wrote and recorded a song and put it on iTunes. It's called "Kayden's Joy," and it is a song I wrote for a charitable project I was a part of. Check it out, it's a labor of love and I couldn't have done it without those catalyst moments that reassured me that I could still break barriers even though I'm not the lowest weight I've ever been. Let God do something big with you as you read this devotional. He is doing big things with me, whether I'm big or small. Remember you are accepted, you are forgiven, you are loved.

Sean Algaier
Former Contestant on NBC's
The Biggest Loser, Season 8

DAY 10

Gluttony—
the Sin Nobody's Talking About

*For, as I have often told you before and now tell you
again even with tears, many live as enemies of the
cross of Christ. Their destiny is destruction, their god
is their stomach, and their glory is in their shame.
Their mind is set on earthly things.*

Philippians 3:18-19

Gluttony seems to be the one sin nobody is talking
about. Ministers preach on adultery, fornication, lust,
strife, anger, hate, gossip and lying, but it is very rare to
hear a sermon on gluttony. In fact, I'm pressed to remember ever hearing a message specifically dealing with gluttony. Why? Because it's a hard subject to teach and an
even harder message to receive.

Many church activities center around food consumption. Church leaders know: if you feed them,
they will come. We Christians call it "fellowship." We
don't do drugs, we don't smoke, we don't go out club-
bing, but we can potluck till the cows come home.
We do the buffet line like nobody's business every
Sunday afternoon!

Gluttony comes from the Latin word *glūtīre* meaning "to gulp or swallow," implying that one is eating so fast as to not even taste the food. Gluttony is overindulgence, over consumption, and a misplaced desire for food. When we constantly think and meditate on what we will eat, where we will eat, how much we're going to eat, or we think of ways to hide our eating from others so they won't know how much we are eating, that is a misplaced desire. Food rules our lives. It is better known in God's Word as an "idol."

There are many strongly stated Bible verses dealing with this particular sin, including Psalms 78:18 which says of the children of Israel: "They willfully put God to the test by demanding the food they craved." And from the wisdom of Solomon, Proverbs 23:21: "For drunkards and gluttons become poor, and drowsiness clothes them in rags. "My personal favorite might be Proverbs 23:2 because it pulls no punches: "And put a knife to your throat if you are given to gluttony."

How do we receive victory and freedom from gluttony and food idolatry? Remember 1 Corinthians 10:31: "So whether you eat or drink or whatever you do, do it all for the glory of God." If you can eat your meal to the glory of God with His blessing, you will walk in self-control, victory and freedom.

> *Father, I want to glorify You with my food choices and my portion sizes. I confess that I have sometimes made food an idol in my life. Help me to choose wisely as I seek to be moderate in my eating and avoid the sin of gluttony.*

EXTREME FAITH AND FITNESS MAKEOVER

When you are bigger than the biggest person on *The Biggest Loser*, it's devastating! That's the way I felt every time that show came on my television. I would sit at home watching while everyone else lost weight and I stayed heavy. At 456 pounds, it almost seemed like it was impossible for me to achieve any kind of success. I turned to my faith in God and put all of my fear upon Him. I had two tiny children who needed their mommy and a husband who depended on me, too. I had finally hit rock bottom. I took a leap of faith and tried out for the first season of ABC's *Extreme Weight Loss*.

I poured my heart out and really leaned upon God and I got picked for the show! I lost a total of 201 pounds over one year, all at home. I met Laurie Graves at the filming for my "big reveal" at the end of the show. Laurie was introduced as a personal trainer who could help me continue on my journey. I was very overwhelmed, and it took me a few weeks to take her up on her offer. Once I did, I knew that I had made the right decision. She is a woman of devoted faith and takes time to carve out a fitness plan for each individual client. She helped me form fitness routines and workout groups for ladies that were just like me—women who still had weight to lose.

I had to have emergency major abdominal surgery in December of 2011 and have since gained back nearly 70 pounds. Laurie has offered me a spot in one of her weekly faith and workout groups to help me continue on where I left off. It's very easy to stray from the righteous path and

keep up with my fitness routines without the accountability and the kindness from others. As you read this
devotional, receive strength and courage. It is possible to
obtain health and move from where you are right now
to a place where you feel more confident. These readings
will give you the strength to see that a journey is before
you and God is certainly there to help you along the way,
even if you stumble!

Staci Birdwell
Appeared on Season 1
ABC's *Extreme Weight Loss*

DAY 11

Be Who God Called You to Be

*I praise you because I am fearfully and
wonderfully made; your works are wonderful, I
know that full well.*

Psalms 139:14

Throughout history there have been different standards of beauty for women. In Renaissance times, white mounds of lumpy flesh were revered as symbols of wealth and status. The Victorians wore tight corsets to emphasize their tiny waists. In the 1950's, Marilyn Monroe was a curvy size 12 and ruled the roost. Every woman idolized her and every man desired her. The 1960's brought Twiggy, the skeletal-thin model who had ladies going on extreme diets to achieve her look. In the late 1970's, Farrah Fawcett showed us that big hair and long legs were the epitome of beauty. Madonna drove the underwear-as-outerwear craze with a heightened sense of overt sexuality in the 80's. And in the last few years, Beyonce' and Kim Kardashian are bringing voluptuous curves back into popularity. Is it any wonder women are confused about body image?

The marketing of beauty and sex appeal affects men, too. Men are told they have to be tall, with wide shoulders, six-pack abs and an amazing car to transport that fabulous body of theirs if they want to measure up.

Society will always try to dictate who you should be. It is Satan's plan to pick you off with negative feelings, unhealthy emotions of unworthiness, and self-condemnation so that you will not step out with confidence to use the gifts God has given you and share them with others for His glory.

Here are four steps to help combat these deceptions of the enemy:

1. Confess with your mouth that you are made for God's glory.
2. Believe that you are wonderfully made by God.
3. Replace negative thoughts with positive ones based on God's Word.
4. Memorize scriptures to combat the enemy's lies.

One of my favorite quotes is by St. Catherine of Siena who said, "Be who God called you to be and you will set the world on fire." Have confidence that God did a good work when He created you and celebrate the beautiful, unique individual He created you to be.

> *Lord, thank you for making me just the way I am. I know you have a special plan and purpose for my life that only I can fulfill. Help me not to get caught up in the world's idea of beauty, but to keep my focus on You.*

FIT FOR FUN IN RETIREMENT

The reason my wife Esther and I attended the Fit for Freedom Challenge was to be motivated to remain active, as I'm retired and she will be soon.

I believe that most of the men in the challenge wanted and needed more accountability. I did lose a few pounds, but the awesome thing was that I went from a 36" waist to a 34."

The best part of class for me was the testimonies. I know I need to commit to regular strength training. For me personally, it's about taking small steps in the right direction. My wife and I are eating better and feeling better already. Thanks for what you are doing for so many of us!

In Christ,
Larry Turner

DAY 12

Think Like a Winner!

*And having disarmed the powers and authorities,
he made a public spectacle of them, triumphing over
them by the cross.*

Colossians 2:15

Can you imagine the battle that took place in the belly of the earth between Satan and our Savior during the three days between Jesus's death and resurrection? Jesus whipped the devil and then according to Colossians 2:15, made an open show of His defeated foe. You know the angels and saints must have been having the party of all parties that day in heaven!

As a follower of Christ, the same power that defeated Satan resides in you. So when you look in the mirror, why do you say you are a failure? Why do you say you'll never amount to anything? Why do you say you'll never be able to get healthy? Why do you tell yourself you'll never be able to stick to an exercise program? Why do you say you'll never be able to have success in your life?

Begin to see yourself as victorious! Jesus gave you the authority to keep the enemy under your feet. He not only defeated Satan, but gave you the Holy Spirit to empower you and help you have daily victory over the enemy.

Meditate on this scripture and know that there can be victory every day for you no matter what your circumstances are:

> **2 Corinthians 10:3-5:** For though we live in the world, we do not wage war as the world does. The weapons we fight with are not the weapons of the world. On the contrary, they have divine power to demolish strongholds. We demolish arguments and every pretension that sets itself up against the knowledge of God, and we take captive every thought to make it obedient to Christ.

We may be fighting an enemy that we can't see, but we *can* see what happens when we relinquish to Satan the power that was handed to us because of Jesus's death and resurrection. So the next time you feel those weak, defeated thoughts start to come up in your spirit, take them captive. Refuse to give the enemy the pleasure of making you think like a loser. Because of what Christ did on the cross, you are a winner. It's time to live victoriously!

> *Thank you, Jesus, for dying on the cross so that I could live in victory. I will claim that victory each day in gratitude for your sacrifice. Help me to take my every thought captive and make it obedient to your will.*

LOSING OVER 400 POUNDS

My name is Earl Ray Kennedy. I'm from Hennepin, Oklahoma. I've always struggled with my weight. All my life, I was made fun of and picked on and had no self-esteem at all. I hid behind my secret walls.

My size was an advantage when I got the chance to live out my childhood dream of becoming a professional wrestler after I graduated from high school. I was trained by the late "Gentleman" Chris Adams and Kevin Von Erich. I loved it! Wrestling was an escape from the real world—and oddly, although the wrestling wasn't "real," I felt I could finally be my real self. After an injury in 1992 left me on the sideline, I became depressed and gained more weight.

In early 1995, I met Stacie, who is now my wife. She had a five month old boy when we met, which I later adopted. Our daughter McKenzie Erin Kennedy was born on March 20, 2000. McKenzie had a heart defect called atrial tachycardia which caused her to have seizures. In September of 2001, I was injured on the job and was unable to work. Depression set in because I couldn't support my family and it was compounded by my concern for McKenzie. I gained to over 900 pounds in no time—913 pounds to be exact!

One day I saw Joyce Meyer talking on TV and she said, "Stop complaining about what you don't have and what you can't do, and think about the what DO HAVE and what you CAN do. Quit having that poor me attitude!" That was the first kick in the pants I received on my weight-loss journey.

Six years later, I had a surge of determination and was able to get down to 720 pounds by myself. I went into a skilled nursing facility and through physical therapy got down to 584 pounds. I was released from the nursing facility in March, 2008 and was able to keep the weight off for about ten months.

Then on January 24, 2009, McKenzie had a spell with her heart and was without oxygen for over 40 minutes. They flew her to Children's Hospital in Oklahoma City. She suffered severe brain damage due to lack of oxygen for so long. McKenzie was on life support for six days. She was trying to fight back early in the week, but on that seventh day, she rested in the arms of God.

My wife and I struggled for some time. I gained to over 770 pounds during that dreadful summer. Just over a year after McKenzie's death, I underwent sleeve gastrectomy. I now weigh 484 pounds—a weight loss of 429 pounds so far since my heaviest weight. For the first time since October 1993, I'm under 500 pounds. Praise God!

In May 17, 2010, I had the chance to attend *The Biggest Loser* season 10 first episode taping in Oklahoma City where I met Bob Harper and the casting producer, Barbara Wulff. I told them my story. Even though I have had the surgery, I still struggle with food every day. It's a constant battle, whether I'm happy or sad. When I am happy, I want to celebrate with food. When I am sad, I want to console myself with food. Overeating is an addiction and I used to be addicted! Food was my drug.

I met Laurie Graves over a year ago, and I can't say "thank you" enough to one of the most thoughtful people I've ever met. Just like God sent me Joyce Meyers to get me motivated, God sent another kick in the pants by way of Laurie Graves. She has put her heart and soul into helping me on my journey. Laurie took me under her wing and taught me to reach for my goal of being a contestant on *The Biggest Loser*, Season 12, even though I was cut at the last minute. I believe in angels and I believe

Laurie is one of a few that have been sent to guide and help me along the way. She accepts me for who I am and has never judged me for my size. She puts me through intense workouts and helped me realize all the things I can do with my 500-pound body. I am grateful for her coming into my life and being another kick in the pants. I officially named Laurie Graves as my trainer on the journey to *The Biggest Loser* season 12 and I am grateful every day that I did!

It is my desire to inspire anyone who will listen to my story. I used to weigh 913 pounds and God has delivered me! If He did it for me, He can do it for you, too! Listen to what Laurie says in this devotional and think like a winner!

Keep moving,
Earl Kennedy

DAY 13

Die to Live

I have been crucified with Christ and I no longer live, but Christ lives in me. The life I now live in the body, I live by faith in the Son of God, who loved me and gave himself for me.

Galatians 2:20

Consider all the pain that Jesus went through during His scourging and crucifixion to give us the power to triumph over temptation, addictions, illness, and negative thoughts. Think about how His flesh was mutilated and ripped open. After suffering an unimaginable beating He still had to endure the crown of thorns, the crowd spitting on Him, Peter's betrayal, and carrying His cross to Calvary. All this suffering was for you.

Jesus fought for your salvation, healing and deliverance, and He defeated the enemy. Because of His sacrifice, you have already won the battle! In order to move from a place of defeat to receiving your victory, you have to lay your flesh down and crucify it daily. You must die to live. You need to decide that you no longer going to accept the temporary comfort that the devil is offering you, and instead utilize the power of the Holy Spirit that allows you to live a wholly victorious life.

With the help of the Holy Spirit, you can say, "Not today, devil! I will not listen to you and drown my sorrows in a whole pan of brownies." "I'm not going to drink my troubles away." "I refuse to pop pills to ease my pain." "Today, I will choose the power of the Holy Spirit and let Him live on the inside of me. He is my Comforter!"

Remember that in order to live—truly live—you are going to have to say "no" to your flesh. And you can do it! The same Spirit that raised Christ from the dead dwells in you if you are a believer. In Romans 8:11 we read, "And if the Spirit of him who raised Jesus from the dead is living in you, he who raised Christ from the dead will also give life to your mortal bodies because of his Spirit who lives in you."

Since Christ is living in you, you have unimaginable reservoirs of strength. You just have to tap into them. Begin living your disciplined life today!

> *Thank you, Lord Jesus, for your sacrifice and your suffering. I give You control of my life. Holy Spirit, be my Comforter as I face the challenges today brings. I will walk in the victory that is mine through Jesus Christ.*

GOD'S GREAT PLAN

I always look forward to going on vacations, whether it's with the family, or the annual "man trip" my buddies and I do every year. I get my gear out and pack, making sure that I have everything—my camera to record memories, bug spray, sunscreen, and enough of the correct clothes for the location that I attend to visit. I get all this together and I am totally psyched.

Recently I was in vacation prep mode when it hit me: why do I get so excited, and do so much planning and prep work to make sure I have the best vacation possible, when I put so little effort into my everyday routine? Why can't I get this excited about having a better, healthier life every day of the year? Face it, if I wanted to go to a theme park, I wouldn't fit on most of the rides, if any at all. Then I thought how sad that would be if my kids wanted me to ride with them, and I had to explain to them that I could not fit in the seat.

My journey with the fitness challenge has made me ask more questions than I have answers for. It has challenged me in many different ways, besides just the weight loss. The one thing that really stands out the most is inviting my Heavenly Father with me on this journey. Whether it is to be still, and listen, or to engage in His Word, I know I can't do this alone. A part of me has to die in order for there to be new life.

Since I have a wonderful wife, a 16-month-old son, and a baby girl on the way, I know that whatever habits I have developed must be changed if I'm going to be the kind of husband and father I want to be. I know I didn't get this way over night, and this journey doesn't stop after I lose about 150 pounds. It's a journey that will take a lifetime, and with God's hand in mine, I know I can move mountains and conquer anything in my way.

I have had spiritual battles with this, in the last twelve weeks, and I have seen God's love for me pull me out of each and every one of them. Also important has been the encouragement of my wife and her allowing me to have some time to myself to work out. Eating right has been a blessing in itself. Traveling as much as I do for work, exercise and a healthy diet are such a challenge.

I have not lost the 25 pounds like I thought I would, but God has a different path for me. I don't know what it is, but I can assure you that if God is in control, and He is, it must be GREAT!

I know I am not perfect, and I will fall, but I will get up, and do it again with God by my side.

Thanks again for your time,
teachings, and your prayers,
Troy Maxwell

DAY 14

Diet vs. Self-Control

But the fruit of the Spirit is love, joy, peace,
forbearance, kindness, goodness, faithfulness,
gentleness and self-control.

Galatians 5:22–23

Over the years I have tried every kind of fad diet out there, only to fail. But through this process, I've learned two important things: 1. Diets are based on the world's wisdom. 2. They usually involve a lot of hype.

There are downsides to nearly every diet plan. For instance, high protein diets work on the principal of dehydration. You lose weight fast, but the weight you lose is mainly water weight. On this type of diet you are generally encouraged to reach "ketosis" which can be very taxing to your kidneys in the long term. The Weight Watchers program, on the other hand, encourages balanced eating. You can eat whatever you want as long as you stay within your daily allotment of "points." This is a great idea in theory. In practice, however, many people store up their points all day so they can overindulge in yummy little cakes at night.

I believe God has a better plan for His children and it's called "self-control." You may be thinking, "Well, Laurie, you don't know me. You don't know my personal struggles. I've tried every diet there is and I do great for a little while, then I fall flat on my face. I just don't have any willpower."

My question to you is: have you tried God's power? Many of us don't even think of approaching a healthy way of eating or our weight loss efforts with God in mind. We grit our teeth and decide we're going to gut it out. We are determined to do it all on our own.

Our Father God cares about our health. He wants us to lay our burdens down and receive His peace and His rest. He even invites us to learn from Him. Diets can be restrictive and lead us to bondage and condemnation. Self-control is empowering. No food is off-limits if we eat it in moderation.

The Greek meaning of self-control is "possessing power; strong; having mastery of." That's what I want—mastery over my impulses. I want to be strong and I want to possess power when temptation comes knocking on my door. Is that what you want, too?

Here is how you do it. Pray this simple prayer when you sit down to meals: *"Father, will You be glorified in this choice and will You be glorified in this portion?"* When you hear yes to both questions, you will be eating with self-control!

NO LONGER ISOLATED AND DEPRESSED

I moved to a new area two years ago, after living in a small community where I had many close friends. In my new town, I was unable to form close bonds of friendship, even at the church I attended. I had become isolated and sedentary, eating my way up to 206 pounds. I am 65 years old, and have been fairly active in the past, but things had settled into non-activity and over-eating. I have previously enjoyed very good health, but my physical check-up in 2011 warned that some areas in my blood tests were elevating to unhealthy levels—not a surprise. My joints hurt to the point that I dreaded going shopping, as the walk through a store was quite taxing.

I know many people who have succeeded in losing weight and keeping it off with Weight Watchers. I went to a meeting, but I knew I could not make that work for me. I can recite the caloric content of every piece of food I see, but that doesn't helped me lose one ounce. I knew I needed something to help me address a life change.

Then quite by accident, someone pointed out the fitness challenge at Northwood Church, and I dropped by that first Saturday. The approach was comprehensive: better eating, changing one's thinking, and moving—EQUALLY important.

The Fit for Freedom Challenge took the subject of overeating much further than calorie counting. Laurie Graves conducted the weekly meetings, teaching on a wide variety of topics from organizing your pantry to organizing your spirit. Laurie had first-hand experience with all the problems associated with her own obesity, and she had gone through the journey of regaining her own health. She is a beautiful person, both physically and spiritually. She understands all the aspects of the challenge—nutrition, exercise, and healing—that God has waiting for everyone.

I have lost 20 pounds so far. I'm not hungry all the time, and I'm not just waiting to get off a darned diet so I

can eat like crazy again, which has always been my thinking in past weight loss attempts. I feel this way of life will
be enjoyable for all the years I will be given. Starving is
not a solution for good health.

Later in the program, I had the wonderful opportunity to work with Laurie to increase my strength and car-
diovascular abilities. No longer sedentary, I pursue daily
activities now that were not possible for me before this
program. I am stronger, able to enjoy a 2-mile walk with
my husband and dog every evening, even adding one
evening per week walking some serious hills in the area.
My latest blood work showed that every single category is
in normal range (even that pesky cholesterol). My blood
pressure is perfect, my blood sugar is perfect, everything
is in alignment. As a senior citizen, I am the Poster Girl
for a perfect blood panel!

Even more than that, I have found people who are
like-minded in their pursuit of good health through the
love of God. Perhaps I have added years to my life, no
one can tell that. But I know the quality of my time is
greatly improved. I had taken a hard look at my future
and saw a dark path of obesity, isolation, pain, depression
and despair. I can't picture any of those in my life now.
God does not want his children to experience that, and
I thank Him every day for gently pointing me to the fitness challenge earlier this year.

Some people who came to the first meetings could
not continue for a variety of reasons, but I know for a fact
that others changed their lives dramatically, and I was one
of those people. There were other ladies with me at those
meetings who were also isolated, obese, and depressed.

How can that be, in our culture of abundant blessings? The enemy is clever, but God heals.

Thanks for everything.

Best regards,
Nancy Anson

Update: This note was recently received from Nancy: "A few months after the Fit for Freedom Challenge, I had unexpected health issues. I am positive that Laurie's fitness philosophy helped me through pneumonia and a serious reaction to an antibiotic. I knew I would get well and pick up my routine again. I have no idea how I could have handled it if I not been strong in body, mind and soul. Since we cannot know what will come to us, I believe we should try very hard to stay as healthy and happy as we can? I've resumed my 2-mile-a-day walk, and rejoice every day."

DAY 15

Return to Sender

Which of you, if your son asks for bread, will give him a stone? Or if he asks for a fish, will give him a snake? If you, then, though you are evil, know how to give good gifts to your children, how much more will your Father in heaven give good gifts to those who ask him!

Matthew 7:9-11

Did you know that God's desire for you is that you live a healthy, happy, abundant life? Many people are experiencing physical pain and suffering and don't understand why. Often, I hear people say, "I believe that God gave me this disease." Or they say, "I believe God is trying to teach me something through this illness." My question to them is, "Then why are you trying to get better? Why visit a doctor and take medicine to get well if you believe that God gave you that disease? If that's truly the case, shouldn't you be embracing sickness to get the full benefit of it?"

I believe God gives good gifts to His children. However, our enemy Satan is constantly looking for open doors to attack us and steal those gifts. In John 10:10 Jesus says, "The thief comes only to steal and kill and destroy; I have come that they may have life, and have it to the full."

Sickness and disease do not sound like full, abundant life to me. I want to believe God for something better.

When the enemy steals the good gifts of health and happiness that our Father in Heaven has given us, he often replaces them with sickness and depression, hoping that we won't do anything about the switch. Ignorant of the truth of God's Word, we unwittingly accept these gifts of disease and infirmity. Don't do it! Mark those false gifts "Return to Sender" and ask God for your complete healing! James 4:2 says, "You have not because you ask not." Seek God's best for your life!

Tomorrow we will address some questions that you need to consider when the enemy knocks on your door with disease or illness, and we will explore biblical answers to those questions.

> *Father God, please give me the wisdom to recognize when I am being attacked by the enemy. Help me to repel those attacks with the shield of faith. Thank you that you have given me a powerful sword of the spirit, Your Word, to protect myself.*

SPIRITUALLY LIGHTER

Thanks for such a dynamic program! I have so enjoyed my Fit for Freedom journey. I feel very good inside and feel confident that I can reach my health and spiritual goals. I am enormously grateful for the valuable growth I have been blessed to receive.

I have a small cyst on my pancreas (which is benign, praise God), but at first the diagnosis had caused me to worry and not be the person I used to be. So I can relate with all the guest speakers who taught on having a proper spiritual mindset. Since entering the fitness journey I have been witness to spiritual healing of my relationships and I have gained a new perspective on life. Gosh, it is amazing! I feel so much lighter now!

We have almost eliminated all those boxed instant dinners and replaced them with better food choices, too!

Sincerely,
Esther Turner

DAY 16

Five Questions on Your Road to Good Health

Do not be wise in your own eyes; fear the Lord and shun evil. This will bring health to your body and nourishment to your bones.

Proverbs 3:7-8

Many times we just look at our illness itself and not the possible root causes of our health problems. When you are faced with a difficult diagnosis, take a minute to go through this list of questions and ask the Holy Spirit to reveal truth to you so that you can take care of any spiritual roadblocks that might hinder you from receiving your healing.

1. **Do I need to repent of sin in my own life so that I can receive my healing?**

   James 5:14-16 says, "Is anyone among you sick? Let them call the elders of the church to pray over them and anoint them with oil in the name of the Lord. And the prayer offered in faith will make the sick person well; the Lord will raise them up. If they have sinned, they will be forgiven. Therefore, confess your sins [my emphasis] to each other and pray for each other so that you may be healed. The prayer of a righteous person is powerful and effective."

2. **Do I have unforgiveness in my heart? Am I holding onto past hurts that are causing bitterness or anger to create problems in my body?**

   Colossians 3:13 encourages us in this way: "Bear with each other and forgive one another if any of you has a grievance against someone. Forgive as the Lord forgave you."

3. **Do I lack wisdom and knowledge on the subject of healing? Do I need to learn more about the cause and prevention of my illness?**

   James 1:5 tells us: "If any of you lacks wisdom, he should ask God, who gives generously to all without finding fault, and it will be given to him."

4. **Have I let cares and worry rob me of sleep and succumbed to stress-related illness?**

   Psalms 4:8 reminds us to trust our Heavenly Father: "In peace I will lie down and sleep, for you alone, Lord, make me dwell in safety."

5. **Have I been disobedient to do the things I've felt God prompt me to do?**

   Exodus 15:26 promises: "If you listen carefully to the Lord your God and do what is right in his eyes, if you pay attention to his commands and keep all his decrees, I will not bring on you any of the diseases I brought on the Egyptians, for I am the Lord, who heals you."

Thank you, dear Father, for providing all the answers I need in Your Word. Help me to be obedient to the direction and wisdom I find there

LOSING CONTROL

Growing up, I was fairly athletic, in good shape and even joined the Army as a young woman. I prided myself on being able to keep up with the guys on the long distance runs. One of my finer moments was running with the unit flag for an eight-mile run when I started my advanced training, not giving it up or quitting when others would try to share the burden of carrying it.

Fast-forward fourteen years from that day and life looked a lot different. I was 35 years old with a beautiful daughter, great husband, a wonderful church and progressing career, but physically I was suffering. Trying to balance it all using my own strength was wearing me out. Running from activity to event, grabbing food on the fly and not taking time for exercise made me a physical wreck. I had gained 70 lbs from my trim Army days. Feeling good about my physical health was a distant memory. Sleep was elusive, as my mind could not relax from the pace of the life I'd been living. There was a point I resignedly said to myself, "So this is how the rest of my life will be." Desperately seeking to be more and do more, I had been living each day in my own strength, and my strength was failing.

Through the providence of God I had a fantastic opportunity to work with Laurie on a 4-week *Losing IT* competition at our church. Because this was a church event, the competitors had the luxury of the accountability of 2500 of our fellow church members to make sure we were making progress. Since Laurie was giving us so much of her time, energy and emotion, I agreed to submit to whatever she recommended for those four weeks and set aside my own agenda. I lost a bunch of weight, over 30 pounds, but more importantly, I lost control. Actually, I didn't lose it. I gave it away—to God.

The Bible says in Proverbs 19:20-21, "Listen to advice and accept discipline, and at the end you will be counted among the wise. Many are the plans in a person's heart, but it is the LORD's purpose that prevails." Though I entered this journey with the intent of getting healthy physically, the Lord's purpose was greater, and His purpose did prevail. He has opened my eyes again to His will for me. Being so busy with activities without the time to properly feed my body or soul is no longer enough! God wants so much more for me than what I can see with my physical eyes, but He will only unfold it when I've taken the steps towards Him.

Whether you are 20 years old or 70, God's not through with you yet! It's no accident that this book was written, or that you chose this book and are reading these very words right now. God is pursuing you to do more and be more through His strength and not your own. "For God is working in you, giving you the desire and the power to do what pleases him," Philippians 2:13.

Dawn Zieger

TAKING STEPS OF FAITH TOWARD FORGIVENESS

Forgiving our offender can be hard, but the journey can start when forgiveness is extended by faith.

Many times we don't feel like forgiving, we don't want to forgive, but I can promise you that when you release and forgive by faith, God can do a HUGE work in YOUR life. If you have identified a person, event or entity (such as a church, business, or organization) as the source of your wound, muster up the courage to say this prayer by faith:

> Dear Father,
>
> You know how _____ hurt me. You know what he/she/they did and You know I've been holding on to the hurt and it's eating me alive. Today, I choose to take a step of faith and forgive. I forgive _____ by faith in Jesus's name for _____ _____. I forgive him/her/them for what he/she/they did to me.
>
> I choose to release _____. They never have to make it up to me; they never have to make it right. I ask you to keep reminding me to release and forgive each time memories of that pain try to rise up in my mind. Your word says to forgive 70 times 70 and I know that there will be opportunities that the enemy will use to bring up this situation again. Help me to be strong enough to forgive again and again.

If your offender is still living:

As an act of my reliance on You and your son Jesus, I bless _____. I bless him/her/them to become all that you have for them. I bless them to come to know Christ in a personal and intimate way. I bless them to be lead on a journey to a closer relationship with You. I bless them to become the man/woman/organization/business/church that You have called them to be.

I am free, in Jesus's name, Amen.

Scripture References

Luke 23:34: And Jesus said, "Father, forgive them, for they do not know not what they are doing."

Matthew18:21-22: Then Peter came to Jesus and asked, "Lord, how many times shall I forgive my brother or sister who sins against me? Up to seven times?" Jesus answered, "I tell you, not seven times, but seventy-seven times."

Ephesians 4:32: Be kind and compassionate to one another, forgiving each other, just as in Christ God forgave you.

DAY 17

Do You Need Balance?

There is a time for everything, and a season for every activity under the heavens.

Ecclesiastes 3:1

Ecclesiastes is a book about seeking perspective—about discovering the seasons of our lives. What season are you in? Some have had a season of feasting, abundance, and excess. This season has contributed to weight gain and may have brought on illness. Perhaps now it is time for a season of restraint and planning.

Others have put the needs of loved ones ahead of their own health. If this is you, you need to block out some time for rest, exercise and proper nutrition. You must take care of yourself or you will be unable to take care of others.

There may also be some who have allowed busyness, stress and lack of sleep to rob them of energy. How can you begin to bring that all back into balance?

King Solomon, who wrote the book of Ecclesiastes as "The Preacher," was the wealthiest man who has ever lived. His life was out of balance, too. He says, "I denied myself nothing my eyes desired; I refused my heart no pleasure. My heart took delight in all my labor, and this was the reward for all my toil. Yet when I surveyed all that my hands had done and what I had toiled to achieve, everything was meaningless, a chasing after the wind; nothing was gained under the sun."

This contemplative book reveals the depression that comes from seeking happiness from worldly things. In the Preacher's reflections, we see the world through the eyes of a person who, though wise, is trying to find meaning in earthly, human things. Although he explores almost every form of worldly pleasure, none of it gives him a sense of meaning.

Toward the end of his life, Solomon came to realize that faith in God is the only way to find true meaning and happiness. He concluded that living is futile without the Lord, and encouraged his readers to reverence God and obey Him.

If your life is out of balance, seek God's perfect will today. Take advantage of Solomon's wisdom and learn from his mistakes. Don't wait until you are experiencing anxiety or illness to begin getting your life in order.

> *Heavenly Father, thank you for loving me enough to let me make my own choices. I want to obey and serve You. Help me to make right choices and align my life with Your perfect will.*

JUST WHAT I WAS LOOKING FOR

Have you ever been flipping through a magazine and have one little page change your entire life? Well, my family has! Last January, my family was not only looking for a church home but was also wanting and needing to get healthier, do some exercising and learn more about nutrition. Guess what!? God, being the great and mighty God that He is, answered all our needs in one little article. My husband found a story about Northwood Church where they were having a 4-week sermon series about getting healthy in spirit, soul and body. We not only found an awesome church, we found an awesome personal trainer and teacher who began helping us through the fitness challenge that followed the *Losing IT* series.

Those classes turned into more health classes, healthier eating, more exercise and we found our awesome church to worship our Father and learn of his loving ways. We also found an awesome lifelong friend, Laurie Graves. Her classes and personal insights have brought me closer to God than any other one person in my entire life other than the minister who led me to the Lord in 1989.

God has richly blessed my entire family by bringing Northwood Church and Laurie into our lives, and for that I am very thankful!

Kathleen Toms

DAY 18

Exercise for Every Season of Life

Let us not become weary in doing good, for at the proper time [in due season] we will reap a harvest if we do not give up.

Galatians 6:9

It is very helpful to try to identify your season of life. Think about your circumstances. Are you dealing with loss of relationship through death or divorce? Maybe you are in a season of raising small children and facing the constraints that monumental task puts on your time and energy. Perhaps you have a new job or a project at work that is causing added stress.

Whatever you are dealing with—ongoing illness, depression, injury, fear of exercise, or lack of energy—there can be a starting place for fitness. Don't just keep sitting on the couch hoping something will happen for you. Find an activity that will fit your personality and season in life. Make sure that it's something you enjoy so that it won't be burdensome.

For instance, if you are overweight, have joint pain, a brittle bones or strained ligaments, the pool is the perfect place to get a non-impact workout. If you are dealing with depression, it can be very healing to be out walking in the sunlight. If you have back pain, rather than lifting heavy weights, it's beneficial to use resistance tubing for an appropriate workout that will strengthen your core.

Another helpful hint is to pick something you enjoyed as a child and try it out again. I discovered when I moved to Holland years ago that I still loved biking and I used my bike as transportation there every day. Now, each summer when it gets oppressively hot in Texas, I can enjoy a gentle breeze that keeps me cool as I ride my bike.

Ask the Father to help you find the exercise that is appropriate for the season of life you are in right now. Take encouragement from today's Bible verse and know that if you will sow energy to exercise, you will reap more energy to be able to perform all the duties you are responsible for *and* you'll have some left over to bless the kingdom of God with!

> *Father God, I don't want to be slothful. Help me to find the right activity to get the exercise my body needs. Let me make good choices so I can be a blessing to my family and others in Your kingdom.*

PEACE IN EVERY SEASON

I have seen myself as fat my whole life. The reality is that I was a healthy weight until after I graduated from high school. I don't know where the unrealistic self-image or poor self-esteem came from. I have listened to the testimonies of pain in people's lives and it is easy to see why people turned to food, but I don't have a story of great tragedy or turmoil in childhood. I can only imagine that Satan knew that he didn't have to surround me with pain because I would beat myself up without much encouragement from him.

In 2007, I joined Weight Watchers and lost 60 pounds in 6 months. I thought I had changed my life forever. I was so focused that I couldn't imagine anything that would cause me to gain the weight back. I met my husband, Troy, in 2009. He had also had success at Weight Watchers and we started out as a great support to each other, but after we were married we had a "food honeymoon" that lasted several months, and we both were gaining weight quickly. During this time, I began hormone treatments for fertility problems. The medications coupled with the stress and fear of not being able to get pregnant brought on more weight. Thankfully, I gave birth to a beautiful son and am now pregnant with our second baby, but I still have the weight to deal with.

In January 2012, I began to increase my exercise and make positive changes in my eating habits. Prior to *Losing IT,* I lost 9 pounds. I joined the Fit for Freedom Challenge primarily to support my husband. I was expecting a food and exercise plan to be given and I knew my foods couldn't be restricted and I wasn't going to be able to exercise intensely because of my pregnancy. Surprisingly, I have been able to fully participate!

The spiritual part of this challenge has been amazing. I have made positive changes in nutrition and exercise, but almost every change has resulted from spiritual guidance which is very new for me. In the past, I have prayed about my weight and I've prayed for self-control but I realized that through it all I was still relying on my own strength. The teaching from Acts 10 on freedom in eating has changed my perspective completely. I connected with the testimonies of avoiding family gatherings and I've been guilty of dictating where and what we ate. I have freedom to enjoy dining with my family and friends now. One of the most important things I learned was how shame and guilt related to food was working against me. When I overate or ate poorly, I somehow believed that I was guilty, and feeling shame was my punishment. Now, I have a new freedom related to food. I'm making better choices, and don't have as much condemnation when I mess up.

I tried to increase my exercise, but have had challenges to overcome. I have incorporated some of the exercises that I can do while doing dishes and folding clothes, etc. I tried to increase my walking, but I found myself very frustrated because my one-year-old would refuse to stay in the stroller for more than 10-15 minutes. I found myself upset with my son and frustrated that I was "trying" to work out and it wasn't happening. One of the testimonies was about having exercise be a time of praise. I realized on a frustrating walk that my attitude was not one of praise and that my son and I were not getting anything positive from our walks. I told the Lord that I was going to praise Him no matter what the length of the exercise. I asked the Lord to bless the time I was able to walk and I know that He has. After a few weeks, my son has become more cooperative about staying in the stroller and I was able to increase my walking time. Now I have a new challenge—when I walk, I have contractions, so I've had to slow my pace way down. Again, in the past, I would have become frustrated and seen this as a setback, but instead I'm trusting that God will honor my efforts and I'm satisfied with what I'm able to do at this time.

My body changes have been minimal, but considering that I am 5 ½ months pregnant I am pleased with the changes in my body and I am thrilled with what I've learned through the fitness challenge.

- First 4 weeks of the challenge: lost 4 pounds
- Final 8 weeks of the challenge: maintained 4 pound loss
- Starting blood pressure: 120/80
- Final blood pressure: 110/70

Thanks, Laurie!

Jennifer Maxwell

Update: Baby Jillian is a healthy, happy toddler. Jennifer has lost all of her baby weight and is working getting to her goal weight.

DAY 19

Write the Vision

*Write down the revelation and make it
plain on tablets so that a herald may run with it.
For the revelation awaits an appointed time;
it speaks of the end and will not prove false. Though
it linger, wait for it; it will certainly come and will
not delay.*

Habakkuk 2:2

Habakkuk was a man determined to get an answer from God. When God answered him, He directed Habakkuk to WRITE. The King James Version of the Bible says, "Write the vision and make it plain." Could it be any simpler than that?

It is a proven fact that when you write down specific goals you are going to be far more successful in weight loss and reaching your fitness goals than the person who has very abstract goals. For example, abstract goals would be general statements such as "I need to lose weight," "I need to get healthy," I should stop smoking," or "I really ought to exercise."

A better way to list goals is to be specific: "I will drink 8 glasses of water a day." "I will walk 3 times a week for 30 minutes." "I will stretch every morning for 10 minutes to gain more flexibility." A successful way to reach your health goals is to journal what you eat, write down emotions that you feel during the day and create an exercise log.

This verse also says that God's revelation will not prove false. The answer you are waiting for—the direction that you need from God concerning your health and wellness—is waiting to come to you. When it arrives, it won't be a lie because the answer and wisdom will have come from God. It will be impressed upon you by the Holy Spirit.

Sometimes we're tempted to use a $19.99 shortcut to a fit body. Don't fall for that. God has an answer on the way and it won't trick, lie or deceive you like those "quick fixes" do.

Pray today's prayer with me:

> *God, I thank You that You are pointing me in the right direction. I thank You that I have wisdom and that You lead me in the path of fitness that is right for me. As you illuminate that path, I will take the time to write the vision that You have given me so that I have a clear set of reasonable, achievable goals that I can review and that will help me stay on track. I thank You that Your answers to me are truth and You never lie or use quick gimmicks or pressure to deal with me. I will avoid using those same things to reach my goals. Thank You that my answer is on the way and that it will come right on time.*

DREAMING AGAIN

I want to thank you for leading the fitness program at Northwood. I was blessed more than I thought possible. I came looking for some recipes and practical advice, and got more than I bargained for! I had started a weight loss program through my job and thought this would complement it. That program basically taught the scientific impact of poor diet vs. a healthy diet, but nothing about the circumstances that got us in this shape to start with.

I only began the program because I was tired all the time. I learned that because of my extreme food allergies, I was trying to function with virtually no protein in my diet and was dehydrated much of the time. When this was corrected, weight started dropping off and I have lost 38 pounds so far, without exercise.

I had no weight-related health issues—great blood pressure, great A1C, and healthy cholesterol levels—so there weren't really any health reasons to motivate me. I am 47, single, no children, and frankly, I've lived life in a rather invisible way—or so I thought. I've never cared much about appearances. No one was looking at me anyway.

I am a teacher, and I also work with students from refugee families in Fort Worth. I told some of my students that I was having a Nepali family visit my church on Sunday, and asked what would be appropriate food to serve them for lunch. I was told rice, vegetables, and fruit. When I asked about meat, some said chicken was okay, but no beef. Most of these students are Hindu and cows are sacred. But then one piped up, "That's not true. If you know Jesus, you can eat anything." They started to discuss that a bit, and I stated that the goal with food consumption was to eat food that made your body healthy. They commented, "Yes, you have been healthier. You used to walk into school with a big Coke in your hand, and now you bring water bottles and salads." I guess I wasn't as invisible as I thought.

When the program started, you asked us to write down a goal or dream. I didn't do it. I quit dreaming a long time ago and have been just surviving for a long, long time. There wasn't any point in it—nothing ever works out for me anyway. But school is out in another week. I think I will need to figure what my goals are and write them down now. I don't know how this will end, but for the first time in a long time, I have hope.

Thank you for the Fit for Freedom Challenge, and for being obedient to God in doing this and giving us all a glimpse of what life could be.

Many Blessings,
Lynn Ketcher

DAY 20

A Merry Heart is Good for Your Body

A cheerful heart is good medicine, but a crushed
spirit dries up the bones.

Proverbs 17:22

For several years I battled depression and thoughts of suicide. My mental problems kept me homebound and isolated. I didn't want to go out and socialize. It was a struggle just to keep up with my household duties and care for my young daughter.

There were many contributors to my depression. Some were of my own making, some were the influences of others, and some were the result of listening to the voice of the enemy. People would casually (and sometimes maybe not so casually) ask, "How are you today?" When I received that question, I always put a big fake smile on my face and say, "I'm doing well, thank you." I covered up my loneliness and depression pretty successfully.

In the King James translation of the Bible, John 10:10 reads: "The thief cometh not, but for to steal, and to kill, and to destroy: I [Jesus] am come that they might have life, and that they might have it more abundantly." I believe my depression was sent by Satan to steal my joy, kill my spirit, and destroy my will to live. Thankfully, God in His mercy intervened and helped me get my spirit, soul and body back on track so I could begin to enjoy the "abundant life" He promised us in this verse.

What's robbing you of the joy of the Lord? The holidays can be a difficult time for many. Sometimes a change in weather, family obligations, financial stress, or memories of loss through death or divorce can all lead to seasonal and ongoing depression. Whether you are struggling with feeling blue or experiencing depression that seems to be taking over your life, there are some things you can do practically and spiritually to enhance your mood.

The first step is to give the burden of your sorrow to Jesus. He is waiting to help. He asks you to come to Him and lay your sorrow at his feet. "Come to me, all you who are weary and burdened," Jesus says, "and I will give you rest."

> *Lord Jesus, I am tired of feeling this bad. I can no longer carry the crushing weight of my depression on my own. I give the burden of my misery to You. Show me what I need to do to get out from under this heartache and pain.*

FITNESS SURPRISE

I had no idea what I was getting myself into when I asked my husband to purchase Amy and Phil Parham's book after that incredible service we attended during the *Losing IT* series. I simply asked for the book. When my hubby got in the car and added, "I signed you up for the challenge," I said, "What!??" Little did I know that it would be life-changing for me!

When I read about Amy's experiences of always putting herself last, always wanting to be a people-pleaser, having her son, Rhett, diagnosed with autism and how she felt the world was caving in around her—boy, could I relate! She was ME! My son was diagnosed with ADHD, OCD and anxiety disorder exactly six and a half years ago. My youngest son was also born almost 7 years ago. That was when the weight really started packing on.

I had to put the book down and weep for awhile, but then something hit me. It was simple, but profound. If Amy was ME and she could do it, then so could I!

I still battle with things on a day-to-day basis, but at least now I recognize it and I'm able to work through it. Before, I would soothe myself with food. If I was stressed, I would eat. If my son and I were having a bad day (and there were a lot of them), I would eat. If I didn't think I was doing a good enough job at whatever I was doing, I would eat. Food was my relief from the real world. I still battle with this demon every day. I feel myself gravitate towards the kitchen when things get rough and I have to catch myself and re-direct into something more positive and healthy!

If I had not gone the Sunday that former Biggest Loser contestants, Phil and Amy Parham, were there, I would still be at 216.5 pounds. I would still be miserable in my skin. I definitely wouldn't have joined the Fit for Freedom Challenge. And I wouldn't weigh 198 today! I have a long road ahead of me (my goal is 150, but at least I got out of the ugly 200's!), but I know I can do it. Hearing everyone's testimonies and seeing true results from the other challengers, I absolutely know I can do it!

Please know that this program absolutely changed my life! My family sees it. I'm starting to notice small changes that keep me motivated to move forward. I turn 50 in September. I am hoping to lose at least another 15-18 pounds before my birthday. How awesome will that be!

Thanks for everything,
Lisa Burdick

DAY 21

Take Control of
Your Emotions

And provide for those who grieve in Zion—
to bestow on them a crown of beauty instead of
ashes, the oil of joy instead of mourning, and a gar-
ment of praise instead of a spirit of despair.

Isaiah 61:3

How do you deal with debilitating depression? Here are five ways to begin getting your emotions back on track.

1. **Look at what you are eating**. One HUGE help in managing depression is to control your intake of refined sugar and processed foods. The body and the brain are just not designed to accept these foods in mass doses. Sugar has depressant chemical qualities and science says it can be as addictive as whiskey or crack cocaine. Do you ever find your mind wandering, taking inventory of what might be in the pantry...thinking about the ice cream in the freezer...or mentally perusing the goodies waiting for you at the convenience store just a few minutes away? If so, you know what it feels like to be obsessing for some sugar, and I can relate!

2. **Exercise can help**. It releases good endorphins that can bring a feeling of happiness to your brain. I have had many doctor-referred clients that were actually prescribed exercise as part of their medical program. I've worked with individuals ranging from the mildly depressed to bipolar, and in all but one case, the amount of anti-depressant medication the client needed was either reduced or eliminated by participating in regular exercise three times per week for 45 minutes.

3. **Spend time with other people.** The enemy loves to work on our minds when we are alone and feeling sorry for ourselves. Initially, you may have to force yourself to be with others. Attending worship services, Bible study or a small group at your local church is a wonderful way to form meaningful, supportive relationships. Christians are encouraged in Hebrews 10:25 to gather together with other believers. The author of this New Testament book knew that we needed the strength and friendships that form among a body of believers to help us stay spiritually healthy.

4. **Search your heart for unconfessed sin**. 2 Corinthians 7:10 says, "Godly sorrow brings repentance that leads to salvation and leaves no regret, but worldly sorrow brings death." Sin can weigh down your spirit to the point that it feels like death. Remember that God's grace is sufficient for you, so if you confess, He is faithful to cleanse you from your sin.

5. **Check your Word level.** Are you spending the appropriate amount of time with the Father to get His daily message for your life? Neglecting God's Word can certainly contribute to a sense of hopelessness and helplessness.

Thank you, Father, for strengthening and teaching me through Your Word each day. I give my heart and my emotions to You. Use me to bless someone in Your Kingdom today.

A NEW DEFINITION OF SUCCESS

As a teenager, all I could dream about was success. I seriously thought that being successful would make me less consumed with my weight. I thought money, high fashion, and great style would blind people to my flaws. I assumed this would be an effective strategy because I witnessed this phenomenon repeatedly occur in school. I noticed that the girl I genuinely cared about only dated "jerks" with money. So I concluded that if I could be the slightly pudgy "good guy" with money, then I could get the girl. Sadly, this became my focus.

I tried everything! At 15 years old, I attended many real-estate seminars, and convinced my mother to join several multi-level marketing companies because I was too young to be accepted. I assured her I would do all of the work. Looking back, I have to laugh. As a freshman in high school I was already trying to overcompensate for something in my life!

I even tried my hand at a "gangster rap" career, even though I was a church-going, never-seen-a-gun, middle-class kid from the suburbs. The music videos of that time had convinced me that this was the route for me. Not to mention the fact that my high school crush loved gangster rappers. This was plenty of motivation for me!

I didn't realize until deciding to sit down and write my story for this book that most of my major high school decisions were based upon my efforts to get the attention of this one girl. I guess I was more of a traditional teen then I thought!

When I made it on *The Biggest Loser*, Season 10, I thought surely all my prayers were being answered! Now I could lose the weight, feel great about myself, and even win $250,000 in the process. Well, God answered my biggest prayer. I lost the weight –175 pounds to be exact—felt great, and made money as a motivational speaker. I was meeting great people who were successful and inspirational. I got everything I had dreamed and prayed for. You would think I would have been happy right? WRONG! I fell into the deepest depression. I would say that I was in despair, due to the fact that God gave me what I wanted and I still wasn't happy. I no longer had hope that anything could make me happy. I ended up gaining back 212 pounds in less than a year. Despair was in full effect!

During this low point in my life, God showed up in some very unexpected places. One of the people that God worked through was Laurie Graves. At a time when my head was always down, she would call and email me with inspiring words and scriptures. When I thought there was no hope, she showed me hope. During this time I was going through therapy, leaning on family and friends, but I still couldn't see how I could get out of my current situation.

One day, while reading through the Bible, I came across this verse in Romans 9:16, *"It does not, therefore, depend on human desire or effort, but on God's mercy."* I had an "ah-ha" moment! The reason I was not happy even when God gave me exactly what I wanted was because I wasn't focused on the most powerful catalyst of change—God. God is love. God is beyond happiness. He is joy! If my focus was on Him rather than my own human desire or effort then I would become a huge success by default!

I began to realize that everyone has a purpose. I have a purpose, even though I may not yet understand or know what it is. I gained the weight back and went through despair for a reason. I met Laurie for a reason. I'm writing this and speaking to you for a reason. I want to encourage you to focus on God, not the weight, and you will lose the weight. *"Seek ye first the kingdom of God and everything else will be added unto you"* Matthew 6:33.

Aaron Thompkins
Former Contestant on NBC's
The Biggest Loser, Season 10

DAY 22

Satisfied

I will be fully satisfied as with the richest of foods;
with singing lips my mouth will praise you.

Psalms 63:5

Have you ever been sitting on the couch watching TV when suddenly you feel the urge to snack even though you just had dinner half an hour ago? You've had your healthy dinner, but now you just aren't satisfied. You are compelled to look in the refrigerator and then go check the pantry for that salty or sweet fix that your body is craving. One of the pastors at my church confessed he has cravings for the "bad stuff" when he's watching *The Biggest Loser* Why is that?

It is called temptation, my friend. It can be the hardest thing in the world to put down the cupcake and practice discipline. These small things can have a huge hold on us, and the enemy uses that to his advantage. But there is an answer. Sometimes a fast from the foods that your body demands may remove that stronghold from your life.

A fast does not have to consist of total abandonment of food. In fact, the Lord will often lead me to have a fast where I sacrifice meat, sugar and bread as an offering to Him. This makes my meals simple and I gain more time for meditation, worship and reading God's Word. In this case, I have given up things I normally enjoy in my diet, but I am satisfied because of the extra time I'm spending with Him.

How could God move if you sacrificed your noon meal to pray? Could God heal your heart if you laid down the doughnut and spent time with Him in the morning? What might happen if you chose to turn off the TV and pick up your Bible instead of a bag of chips?

Remember the story of Daniel that I shared with you? Because Daniel and his friends refused the king's meat and practiced sanctification and obedience to God, they were strengthened to go through their fiery furnace experience with God's help.

In fact, even faced with death, they were strong! God protected them so well they came out not even smelling of smoke! Did they know that they were going to have such a severe testing of their faith when they chose to eat to please God? No. God was preparing them for upcoming events. Not only did they come out of the furnace unharmed, they were promoted to high positions of authority by the king.

You are preparing for your future when you fast!

> *Lord, I want to put You first in my life. I lay down the food that has a hold on me at the foot of the cross. Work in my heart, Father. Make me the person You want me to be so that I can fulfill the role you have for me in Your kingdom.*

BETTER LATE THAN NEVER

I want to share with you a bit of what your program meant to me!

First off, I want to thank you for being a blessing and life-changer for my kiddos! I'm a much better, healthier mom. I love your program's combination of both physical and spiritual fitness! It's truly "God's way!"

God used you to get me back on track also. In many ways, I'm a "late bloomer." I started my career at 45, got my master's degree at 50, and now about two-thirds of the way through this challenge, I am on track! God's inspiring words through you set me up for a serious talk with my doctor. God used you to prepare my heart to take action on what my doctor told me. Now rather than yo-yoing up and down with my weight, I'm making progress on the road to health and fitness! I've changed from saying and thinking "I'm trying to…" to "I am…"

Once again, I want to thank you for answering God's call!

Blessings,
Marilyn Johnson

DAY 23

Beginning Exercise

Be strong in the Lord and in his mighty power.

Ephesians 6:10

I want to encourage you to stay strong. Don't let anything hinder your decision to work on your health. If you have a friend or family member who will join you, you will be stronger as a team working toward the same goal.

If it's been some time since you've exercised, it's best to start with some walking or swimming. Joints and ligaments can become loose, and by starting out hard and heavy, you may find it causes more harm than good. By walking, you can strengthen muscles, exercise your heart, and train your joints and ligaments to take on more aggressive workouts.

Many of my clients tell me they have pain in their lower back, knees, hips, ankles, and feet when they exercise. Perhaps you do, too. Here is a great reason to get that extra weight off: Did you know that for every pound you take off, you take four pounds of pressure off your joints? If you take off 10 pounds, that's 40 pounds off your joints. If you take off 25 pounds, that's 100 pounds off these key points. And if you lose 100 pounds, you'll have taken a whopping 400 pounds of pressure off these areas of your body that are crucial to normal everyday living!

Do you ever think, "I don't have time to exercise?" Many individuals struggle in the beginning to incorporate exercise into their daily routine due to of lack of time management skills. I believe that God will give you creative ideas to make time for exercising. But remember—you will never just magically have 45 extra minutes in your day to give yourself the gift of health. You are going to have to schedule it in. You'll have to strive for it. It has to be on your calendar and you are going to have to want it because you know that it's your reasonable service to God.

Make exercise a priority in your day. You will feel better physically and mentally, and you will be giving your metabolism and your immune system a boost.

> *Thank you, Heavenly Father, for giving me the ability to exercise. Build in me the desire to do it. Don't let me be a sluggard, Lord. I want to have a strong, healthy body that is pleasing to You.*

BURDENS RELEASED

During the fitness challenge, I lost 15 pounds (which is a dress size!) and was able to get my gluten-free diet under better control. I want to thank you, Laurie, for everything that you did for me. The weight loss was by far the smallest part of the journey I went through over these past 12 weeks. You have inspired me with your humility and graciousness. As a result of your teaching, I have been able to find forgiveness and release burdens I have carried for years.

My journey has truly just begun.

In faith,
Kellie Weir

DAY 24

No Longer in Disgrace

*Then I said to them, "You see the trouble we are
in: Jerusalem lies in ruins, and its gates have been
burned with fire. Come, let us rebuild the wall of
Jerusalem, and we will no longer be in disgrace."*

Nehemiah 2:17

The second and third chapters of Nehemiah tell of
God giving a vision and direction to Nehemiah about a
special task that He had for him to do. Nehemiah was
being sent to repair the walls and gates of Jerusalem. In
those days, if you didn't have walls around your city to
protect it, you were in really big trouble. You were open to
attacks. Your enemies could come right in and take whatever they wanted at any time.

Whenever I read this story, I think of the disrepair
that existed in my own life eight years ago. My walls were
a mess. Because I had no order and no structure to my
life, I was wide open to depression. I had thoughts of
suicide and I had numerous eating disorders. I was wide
open to all the negative thoughts the enemy brought to
my mind because I had no defense system.

Nehemiah knew God had assigned him the task
of repairing the walls. We also know that we have an
assignment from God to keep ourselves in good health.
Hopefully, as you read this devotional you have been

doing the same things Nehemiah did: surveying, assessing, praying and asking God to give you the right plan for your body.

Late one night, Nehemiah went out on a donkey to conduct a survey of the city walls. The donkey could not even navigate the mess of rubble and rocks. Initially, I started tackling my weight loss the same way Nehemiah began his project—in the dark. I didn't want anybody to know what I was doing. I didn't want to tell anyone I was on a diet. After all, what if the job turned out to be too big and I couldn't accomplish the task?

Nehemiah realized that he couldn't do this job on his own—it was just too big. He expressed his need for help and people came from near and far. They came from different social and economic levels, different ages, and different skill levels—all to help repair the walls. Isn't that just like God? He gave Nehemiah a HUGE plan and vision. But all Nehemiah had to do to achieve his dream was step out in obedience and God had people right there to help him. I had lots of help on my journey to good health, too. Trainers, doctors, books, and friends all helped me to reach my goal. Who has God brought to your life to help you rebuild your walls?

God continues to repair the walls of faith and obedience in my life, and I believe it will be an ongoing process as I continue to learn to walk out my healing.

> *Thank you, God, for the vision and the desire to get healthy. Please bring the right people into my life at the right time to help me reach my goal so that I will no longer feel in disgrace.*

SMALL STEPS ADD UP TO
BIG RESULTS

After hearing about the fitness challenge at church one Sunday morning I decided to sign my 18-year-old daughter Salina and myself up. During the first few classes, I just sat there and listened more than anything. Then I decided to start keeping track of the food I was eating to see exactly what it was I was putting in my body. I had no idea that a lot of the time I was just eating out of habit and not even because I was hungry.

I have spent most of my life being overweight and now was passing this along to both of my daughters. My husband and I talked a lot about what I was learning at Laurie's classes and decided as a family to make some lifetime changes. All four of my grandparents had heart issues and so did my dad. I can't fight genetics, but there is something I can do about my weight and the way my family eats.

I started logging in everything I ate and drank into my smartphone and began exercising every other day. Other than my morning coffee, all I would drink was water. I started cooking healthier meals and was amazed at what my family actually enjoyed eating. It's still not the easiest thing to get my girls to eat fish, but I'm working on it.

Over the last month, I have been going to an exercise bootcamp and started a walking club for teachers at my school. I do some kind of physical activity every day. I even found a workout room at a hotel this past weekend when we went out of town. I NEVER thought that would be me. Last March, I had lower back surgery. But since I've lost 33 pounds, my back is no longer a problem! I actually crave water and rarely go a day without exercising. This has truly been a lifestyle change, not just for me, but my entire family. It's one day at a time, but I now look forward to those days more than ever before.

Ashley Ball

UPDATE: Ashley has now lost 70 pounds since the Fit for Freedom Challenge began! She also took the Faithfully FIT and FIT 4 Freedom classes that Laurie offered and she's totally changed the way her and her family eat and exercise. Because of Ashley's decision to get healthy, her whole family has changed—for the BETTER! They are eating together, cooking at home more and exercising together. Just recently Ashley's 9 year old daughter lost 9 pounds and her husband has lost 15 pounds. She and her husband have both shaved 20 points off their cholesterol numbers. When Ashley started doing the things that the Holy Spirit showed her she should do and she took the steps of obedience to do them, she and her family were greatly rewarded. It's a ripple effect!

DAY 25

Let Go and Live!

For I take no pleasure in the death of anyone,
declares the Sovereign LORD. Repent and live!

Ezekiel 18:32

This verse in Ezekiel 18 is set in the 6th century B.C. Israel had been invaded by Babylon. Through Ezekiel, the Lord is giving the children of Israel a warning.

God tells them that that they are going to die for their own sins, not for the sins of others. He tells them, "Stop blaming your parents for your sins. Stop blaming your spouse or your children. Grow up and take responsibility for your own shortcomings. You are going to die because of your OWN sins." Ouch! That's pretty harsh, isn't it?

Many times, I have to tell my clients pretty much the same thing, and now I'm telling you. It's your fault that you eat too much and exercise too little. I know it's hard to hear, but YOU have the responsibility for your own health. God is giving you the opportunity to straighten yourself up and take action so that your spiritual, emotional and physical health does not come to ruin.

"Oh, Laurie," I can hear you say, "I don't want to hear that. I need someone to take responsibility for my problems—someone besides me, of course. It's too hard on my self-esteem to acknowledge that I am the cause of my own problems. It has to be someone else's fault."

I've heard it all before. Many times people blame their current physical problems on offenses they received in the past. "I am the way I am because of my childhood." "My wounds are deep." "You don't know how my mom damaged me." "You don't know what my dad said to me." "You don't know how hard my divorce was." "You don't know how badly it hurt when my friend walked out on me and I've just never recovered."

I'm sorry those things happened to you in the past, but *they happened in the past*. Let it go. By holding on to these offenses you will never be able to walk in freedom. Facing the future while bound, tied and gagged by yesterday sounds miserable, doesn't it?

Do what I've had to do—ask the Father to help you let go of past hurts and release the offense of others so you can be free to be everything God wants you to be. Let go and live!

> *Dear Lord, I don't want to be a victim any longer. I'm willing to take responsibility for my own actions. Help me to let go of the pain that I've been carrying and help me to forgive those responsible so that I can move forward with my life.*

BRING EVERYTHING TO GOD

It is common for believers to unwittingly compart-mentalize our lives, segregating the parts in which we truly involve God from the rest of our lives. Yes, we may ask for His help to get through a rough day at work, to keep us safe as we travel, or to overcome the urge to eat that yummy-smelling doughnut, but then we stick God back in His spiritual compartment and get on with our lives. We may actually believe we are involving God in all aspects of our lives, but how often do we ask Him to come alongside us and really be a partner in our journey?

I grew up in instability. I could never count on much of anything except change. My dad was in the military and he was always gone. When he came back, that usu-ally meant we were moving. I learned to adapt, but to never sink roots. I made friends, but kept an emotional distance from them because I would be leaving soon. I still have a hard time fully investing in people. I have also always endured ridicule for being fat. I am always the butt of jokes. Even the best intentioned people call me "Big Guy" or "Big Man." My solace has always been food. Food is a comfort. It makes me feel good and I can always count on it. Even after I became a Christian, I would run to food long before I would even think to run to God.

To this day, I struggle with my weight and I assume that it will always be this way for me. I sometimes feel as though my weight issues are too trivial to bring to God for help. However, in reality, my weight has been a huge part of my life. Starting from childhood to now I have spent countless hours thinking about it, trying to lose it, trying to hide it, and feeling inadequate because of it. Laurie's book has helped to remind me of how loving and caring the God that we serve is, that He really does care about us, and that He wants us to come to Him with everything (even if it seems trivial). He desperately wants to help us. He *is* our stability and we can *always* count on Him. We just need to remember to keep running to Him instead of to food.

Laurie has helped to lead me toward a better way of looking at the relationship between me, God, and my health. She has shown me that together, God and I can overcome even the biggest problems and He will help me become the best version of myself that I can be.

Thanks a lot, Laurie!

Corey Pinkerton,
Former "At Home" Contestant on NBC's
The Biggest Loser, Season 10

DAY 26

Here We Go Again

*This is what the Sovereign LORD, the Holy One of
Israel, says: "In repentance and rest is your salvation,
in quietness and trust is your strength."*

Isaiah 30:15

Have you ever noticed that when you get one thing
under control in your life, sometimes a new habit or addiction will surface? For instance, when I lost 90 pounds I
finally had my diet in check, but I started shopping too
much. Thousands of people stop smoking, but then gain
weight because they eat too much. Some people give up
drugs, only to start drinking. Why is that?

I believe it has something to do with a lack of repentance. In our culture, we are encouraged to fix our problems without getting anyone else involved. We are taught
to pull up our bootstraps or put our big girl panties on,
and just suck it up. We don't have to admit to being in
the wrong as long as we fix what was broken. That might
work for some things, but in my own life I've found that
my addiction can only be healed in the presence of a
holy God.

Healing occurs when I acknowledge that my body is
the temple of the Holy Spirit. I have to realize that whenever I partake in my addiction, I am forcing the Holy
Spirit to participate in my sin because He lives inside me.

When I have had a repentant heart over the way I've mistreated my temple and the sorrow I have caused the Holy Spirit, I have experienced brokenness and a willingness to change.

When it comes to fitness, most of us want the magic bullet. "Lose 30 pounds in 30 days!" "Get lean, fit and ripped in 90 days!" "Be beach ready in 5 minutes a day!" "Eat your way to skinny!" These infomercial promises can provide short-term satisfaction, but unless you repent and become broken enough to rely on God's strength and His words to carry you, you'll gain weight right back or you'll transfer your sin to another addiction.

Begin your transformation to complete freedom by asking God for forgiveness and healing. Pray this prayer with me.

> *Holy Spirit, thank You for opening my eyes to the root of my sin. I turn from it and I will keep my eyes on You. I am sorry that I have involved You in my addiction. Break the hold it has on me and help me get free from anything that would keep me in the bondage of sin.*

WEIGHT LOST, PURPOSE GAINED

I volunteered as one of the original contestants in Northwood's *Losing IT* weight-loss challenge. It was great, but it wasn't easy. It wasn't like it is on *The Biggest Loser* television show. I didn't get to go to the ranch and focus entirely on losing weight. I had to go to work every day at my job, plus work out twice a day. So there were days that left me exhausted—but no more so than some of my regular days. As I began to lose weight and eat in a new and healthier way, I actually started feeling better than usual. At the end of three weeks I had lost 27 pounds, and I was declared the *Losing IT* winner!

It was an incredible time. I went through a total transformation of body, mind and spirit. One of the things that God taught me during the challenge was the importance of feeding my spirit. Laurie's focus on the spiritual aspect of the program allowed me to hear from God in a way that I hadn't heard from Him in a long time.

One Sunday, I heard that the Vietnamese government had asked my church to help them pioneer a child abuse prevention program for their country. I knew God was leading me to be a part of it. Normally I would have immediately dismissed the idea, saying that I couldn't afford to travel to Vietnam (which was true), or that I wasn't the most qualified person to help in this area (also true). This time, however, I felt the Holy Spirit compelling me to use my skills and abilities as a social worker to help children who desperately needed someone to speak on their behalf, and I knew that God would help me to do it. I decided to step out in faith and commit to being part of the team that would teach Vietnamese medical professionals, social workers and law enforcement agencies how to recognize and intervene in child abuse cases.

My cell group at church, my friends, and even my *Losing IT* buddies helped me to raise the money to go to Vietnam. The Vietnamese people were so welcoming and so appreciative of everything that our team had to share. The best part of all was knowing that children were going to be cared for and protected as a result of what we were teaching the leaders in their country.

I don't know if I would have had the energy or determination to take part in this effort if I hadn't lost the weight. And I don't know if I would have been obedient to the Lord's leading in the first place if Laurie hadn't been insistent that spiritual fitness was just as important as physical health. She taught me that the reason I need to take care of my body is so that God can use me to serve others.

I've lost 8 more pounds, and it's been great, but I've found that even better than being thin is being obedient to the Heavenly Father. It's been an amazing journey so far, and it's just beginning!

Kurt Pafford

DAY 27

God's Words Bring Healing

My son, pay attention to what I say;
turn your ear to my words. Do not let them out of
your sight, keep them within your heart;
for they are life to those who find them and health to
one's whole body.

Proverbs 4:20-22

By applying God's Word to areas of your life that are out of control, you can receive a total healing. Have pen and paper handy and follow these steps.

- Bow your head and ask the Holy Spirit to illuminate truth to you in the moment. Ask the Father to show you the true attitude of your heart right now as you go through this exercise of brokenness, forgiveness and healing.
- Quietly pray and ask the Holy Spirit to show you where the problem lies. Is it a wrong attitude or emotion? Is there a generational habit or addiction that needs to be broken? What changes do you need to make in your life?

- Once the Holy Spirit has illuminated that to you, tell Him you accept responsibility for the sin. Don't blame your behavior on someone else.
- Tell the Father you apologize. Let Him know that you realize you were wrong.
- As an outward representation of your inner commitment to turn from your sin, use your paper and pen to write a word or short sentence that describes the sin you are repenting. When you are finished, tear up the paper and throw it on the floor. Stomp on it if you want.
- Now lift your hands and thank the Father for His healing power. Thank Him that He has delivered you. Continue to praise Him for being your Healer each and every day for the rest of your life. The enemy does not want to stay where God's name is being praised. He will flee.
- Know that the enemy will try to come back. You must resist him and hold him back with the power of God's Word. Speak scripture aloud, read the Word, and meditate on it.

Father God, thank You for being Jehovah Rapha, the God Who Heals. I am in awe of Your power and Your majesty. I can never praise You enough. Take my life and use it for your glory.

MY JOURNEY FROM WORTHLESS TO WEIGHT-LESS

All my life I struggled with my weight. I was the chubby kid, the fat teenager who never got asked to the prom. As a form of self-preservation I became "funny, fat Julie." I used my sense of humor —often in a self-depre-cating way—believing that if I was already laughing at myself, others wouldn't laugh at me.

So it's no surprise that I also became an overweight adult. I yo-yo dieted for years, trying every fad diet that came out. I'd have a little success here and there, but no real lasting change. On the outside I was smiling and laughing, always putting others at ease. On the inside, though, I was uncomfortable in my own skin.

My struggle was magnified because I had given my life to Christ at age thirteen. However, I just couldn't shake the fact that I believed God was *mad at me* for being fat. Everyone else in my life had put "conditions" on their love for me (or so it seemed). Why wouldn't God? A bat-tle with low self-worth seemed to plague me.

In my mid-twenties I married the love of my life. And although I still wasn't happy with my weight on my wedding day, I had managed to starve myself into what I believed was an acceptable size. Soon after we married, the desire for a baby came. We ended up having to go to a fertility doctor and I needed surgery before I was ever able to conceive. But miraculously I did have a precious baby boy. We named him Noah, which means "peace." (And we have had very little of it since he arrived!)

As a mom, I began to pour my whole identity into this little life. He became everything to me. And all the while my weight continued to spiral out of control. With the very best of intentions of putting everyone and everything ahead of myself, I became the last thing on my list of priorities. It all came to a head when my doctor used the term "morbidly obese" to describe me. I was crushed by those words.

You see, five pounds had become ten pounds; ten became twenty. I rationalized all of it, saying I could eventually get it off. But when twenty pounds became one hundred pounds, I didn't know where to go or what to do.

Finally, I cried out to God with a prayer I know I had prayed hundreds of times before, but there was something different this time. I said, "God, if you will just help me…I promise to *finally* make a change."

Shortly after that simple prayer, I received a call from a friend who told me the producers from the reality show *The Biggest Loser* were coming to my hometown. I jumped at the chance to go to a casting call. I had been a fan of the show for years, always believing I could do what I saw others on TV doing. I marveled at the jaw-dropping transformations at the finale each season and I dreamt that one day it could be me!

The casting process was quite tedious. After a year of waiting, I finally got the confirmation that I had been selected to be part of the cast of Season 4 of *The Biggest Loser*. The experience was life-changing to say the least. I have never worked so hard or sweated so much in my life. But it ended up being far more about what I *gained*, than what I *lost*.

God did a transforming work in my life, and He used—of all things—a reality TV show to accomplish His plan for me. As I said, I had always believed God was mad at me for being fat. What I learned through this process is that He wasn't mad *at* me. He was madly in love *with* me. When I finally grabbed hold of that reality in my heart, not just my head, everything changed for me. I truly embraced—for the first time—my value and worth.

One of the main reasons I wanted to be on *The Biggest Loser* was the deep desire to have another child. Health issues associated with my weight had contributed to my infertility diagnosis. After losing nearly 100 pounds (45% of my body weight) I thought conception would be simple! But the Lord had different plans yet again.

Shortly after completing the show and finishing as the "Biggest Female Loser" of the season, coming within eight pounds of winning the actual title, I settled into my new lifestyle and told my husband I was ready to try to have another baby. He shared that God had impressed upon him while I was on the show that we were to adopt a child.

I was skeptical to say the least. But in a series of events that was more miraculous than being selected out of half a million applicants to be on a reality TV show, we brought home a baby less than two weeks after submitting a family profile to a local adoption agency. We named our newborn Jaxon (with an "x"), which means "God has been gracious," which He has.

In addition to the lesson I learned about the enormous worth we all possess as children of God, I also learned a valuable lesson that God's plans are so much greater than our own. If I had won *The Biggest Loser*, I would have been contractually obligated to travel a great deal. And I wouldn't have been free to receive the one gift that I truly wanted the most: a baby. God knew the deepest desire of my heart and He planned the way to fulfill that desire perfectly.

For five years I have worked hard to maintain a healthy weight and lifestyle. And this has been the story I have shared with thousands of people through a ministry as an inspirational speaker: that we all have incredible worth which is placed within us by our loving God, regardless of whether we are fat or thin.

And I believe that with all my heart.

So it was quite a challenge for me when I learned that the infertility diagnosis from years ago was no longer accurate, and at age 40 I was pregnant! Now, you might think that my first thought would be elation —being overjoyed at the thought of having a baby after all those years of infertility. But you see, for a woman who has been on *The Biggest Loser*, it's not quite that simple. Oh, the joy came soon after. But my first thought was: "How can I do this without gaining weight?"

My weight was always my self-perceived greatest weakness. It was the thing I was most ashamed of. But now losing weight is what I am best known for. The question others ask about me most often is: "Has she kept the weight off?" I knew that as my stomach grew, I would face stares from people who wondered if I had "fallen off the wagon."

This pregnancy was different than my first. I started out healthy and although I gained weight, I now have all the tools and knowledge of how to get it off again. I have had to re-remind myself that my value and worth does not come from my size. And that God's plans are so much bigger and better for us than our own.

I realize we all carry unnecessary weights; and some of them have nothing to do with the number on the scale. Finding my worth in the eyes of my Creator was the key to being able to let go of —not just my physical weight— but all of the things that "weighed me down."

I am grateful to God for each step of the journey. It's a wonderful feeling to live the life I believe I was created to live…and to have made the transition from worthless to weight-less.

Julie Hadden
Former Runner-up Contestant on
NBC's *The Biggest Loser*, Season 4

DAY 28

To Sleep, Perchance to Dream

In peace I will lie down and sleep, for you alone,
Lord, make me dwell in safety.

Psalms 4:8

In 1984, the British Medical Journal ran an editorial warning that the hurry and excitement of modern life was leading to an epidemic of insomnia. Imagine where we are today! We are overworked, over-scheduled, and over-committed. You would think that with all that activity we would sleep like babies at night. Yet we toss and turn, unable to get any rest.

Why is lack of sleep so prevalent today? I believe it comes from economic stress and the fear that comes from financial uncertainty, worries about children and relationships, an inability to wind down properly at night, and over-stimulation from all the screens in our life. Television, Facebook, iPads, iPods, laptops and notebooks vie for our eyes and minds 24/7.

Studies over the last 40 years indicate that most adults need 7–7 ½ hours of sleep per night. There are a few people that can function fine with less, but they are rare. Your body can keep going without enough sleep, but your

brain can't. Even missing just one night of sleep impairs
motor function and adversely affects mood. Lack of sleep
makes it harder to cope with stress. We can become for-
getful and even the simplest of conversations can become
difficult when we are exhausted.

Try these practical steps to help you get better sleep
tonight:

- Turn off all screens one hour before bedtime.
- Meditate on the good memories and /or accom-
  plishments of the day.
- Consider keeping a "Thankfulness Journal" where
  you jot down one or two blessings of the day.
- Spray lavender mist in your room or use lavender
  oil on your pillow. It's reported to improve quality of sleep by 20%.
- Pray before bedtime.

Your evening prayer might be something like this:

> *Heavenly Father, I desire to honor the Temple that
> you have blessed me with. I ask you to give me wis-
> dom to turn off the TV and other electronic devices.
> Help me to let go of all the stress of the day and speak
> to me right now. Quiet my soul and bring me peace
> as I trust You through the night. I trust You for
> refreshing sleep so that I can be at my best mentally
> and physically, enabling me to handle the tasks and
> responsibilities on my list for tomorrow. In Jesus's
> name, Amen.*

BEING THE LONE RANGER IS NO FUN

One of the key things for me during the weight loss challenge was being part of a group. I felt that working out with others was crucial to being able to stay on track. Working out alone is no fun. It just feels like work. But having someone else there to encourage you, seeing you struggle and saying, "You can do it!" makes it so much better. And when you see others being successful, you say, "Hey, I want that, too!" So you work extra hard, and that's really cool.

Through this experience, I've developed close friendships and lost 25 pounds. You would think a competition like *Losing IT* would be all about beating the other guy, but it's not. It's about supporting each other and building new relationships, and that's really cool. Now I actually look forward to going to the gym and working out, and that is a miracle!

Brad Zieger

DAY 29

Fighting Giants

David said to Saul, "Let no one lose heart on account of this Philistine; your servant will go and fight him."

I Samuel 17:32

You will find the familiar story of David and Goliath in 1 Samuel 17. The shepherd boy David had been sent by his father to bring food to his brothers who were fighting the mighty Philistine army. David arrived to find that there had been no progress in the battle. In fact, for the past 40 days and nights the Philistine champion, Goliath, had tormented the Israelites by calling out blasphemies against them and their God.

When David witnessed what was going on, he became enraged. He had identified a BIG problem that needed to be solved in order to bring peace and prosperity to his nation and its people. Once he identified the problem, he knew it had to be dealt with. Since no one else had the courage to face Goliath, David decided that with God's help, he would take this foul-mouthed, God-cursing giant down!

He knew that on two different occasions when he was out in the field tending to his sheep God had given him the strength he needed to protect his flock. With God's help, he had killed a lion and a bear. As he recalled those victories, courage and determination rose up in him.

Once he convinced his brothers and the king to let him attempt the thing God had laid on his heart to do, they gave him armor that was too heavy for him. He couldn't move properly, so he left it behind and instead chose to take something he was more comfortable with: a slingshot—a boy's toy—and five stones. He also took the name of the Lord God Almighty.

Can you imagine how his heart was pounding and how his mind must have been racing as he stepped out onto that field and faced Goliath? It was a total step of faith. Running toward the Philistine who was laughing and promising to feed him to the birds, David saw his opportunity. There was an opening in the giant's protection—his helmet left his forehead bare. David aimed right for it and landed a stone so hard it embedded right above the giant's eyes, knocking him out cold. David wasn't going to take any chances. He ran over, pulled out the giant's sword, took total authority, and chopped Goliath's head off.

This is exactly how I have had to approach the giants of depression, rejection, divorce, obesity and a whole host of other enemies that Satan has brought into my life. I have had to identify the enemy, remind myself of past victories, use weapons I'm familiar with, and have confidence that God will deliver me. I know that Jesus has already given me the victory to eradicate every force of darkness that tries to exalt itself in my life. I just have to be willing to fight.

> *Lord Jesus, thank you for giving me the tools I need to battle the giants in my life. With Your help, I will defeat them, and when I do, I will give You all the glory. I am confident in You.*

OBEDIENCE BRINGS AMAZING GIFTS

Working with Laurie Graves during *Losing IT* changed my life forever. Prior to this event, I had worked with Laurie for almost a year. I was losing weight off my body, but not weight off my shoulders. I had worked hard to "do all the right things" and put on a show of sorts to prove I was doing it all, but I forgot the most important ingredient: God.

I thought that I could do it all alone. I was the one who had created this "mess" of my body through over-eating, and I thought I needed to clean it up. Silly me! I thought I had it all together and it was just a matter of eating the right foods and exercising the right amount. Again, silly me!

What I learned during *Losing IT* and the Fit for Freedom Challenge was that the battle was my own, but I did not have to fight all alone. I realized that behind the number on the scale, I was fearful of failure. I was scared to be me. I was afraid to have others see my weakness.

As I stepped on the scale in front of the entire church, a layer of my onion peeled back as I realized I couldn't hide behind a number anymore. My journey had just become public! It was very different from the TV show. On *The Biggest Loser*, they get to leave fat and return home skinny. I showed up every week still fat. I lost weight, but I was far from being thin. What I gained from *Losing IT* and making my journey public was seeing that I can be me and still have support. People were cheering me on, wanting me to succeed.

Losing IT ended and the fitness challenge began, and I really began to change inside. I began to see that I needed a close group of people to form a community that would help me continue on this journey. I realized that just because I had lost a lot of weight and figured out many of my triggers, I still needed a daily journey with God. It became not just my weight-loss journey, but a journey to obedience: obedience to what God has called me to do, obedience to follow directions given in His word, obedience to being the "me" He has called me to be.

After the fitness challenge was over, things in my family continued changing and we were truly working together toward a healthy lifestyle, both physically and spiritually. After four years of missing or extremely long menstrual cycles, my cycles started to shorten and become regular. My husband and I had been trying to have another child for five years, and to my surprise and delight, we are now pregnant! I can only attribute this to my obedience to follow through with what God had called me to do with my body, mind and spirit.

I was hoping to lose more weight to get out of the 'extremely obese' category, but God's timing is perfect and I cannot wait to meet this little blessing! Then we can all continue on this journey of health and obedience together.

Jodi Pafford

Jodi lost 37 pounds during the Losing IT series and the Fit for Freedom Challenge. She and her husband, Kurt, have since welcomed a bouncing baby boy into their family!

DAY 30

Battle Plan

*Then he took his staff in his hand, chose five smooth
stones from the stream, put them in the pouch of
his shepherd's bag and, with his sling in his hand,
approached the Philistine.*

I Samuel 17:40

David approached Goliath with confidence. He knew
that the living God was on his side. You can defeat the
giant problems in your life, too. You just need to have a
battle plan. Here's how to get started:

1. Recognize your enemy. Identify the problem that
   screams and torments you day and night.
2. Choose your armor and weapons wisely. The Word
   of God, prayer, determination, and past victories
   are all weapons of destruction against the enemy.
3. Know your weapons. What's in your bag?

   - When you are tempted to pig out on fast
     food, which of your rocks will you use?
   - When the enemy invites you to sit and watch
     television instead of walking, which rock will
     get you off the couch?
   - When your well-meaning friends encourage
     you to fill up your plate two or three times at
     a picnic, which rock will help you to resist?

- When your family refuses to acknowledge that you are making an effort to lose weight, which rock will stop the sabotage?

Once you have had one successful battle, it gets easier. I know from experience. Once you have had some victories, you'll know how to fight more effectively. David knew which actions needed to be taken and he had the confidence to take them. I pray that by the time you have read through these daily encouragements, you will as well. Get your rocks ready and be prepared to fight!

> *Father God, please help me to recognize the giants in my life—anything that is displeasing to You or contrary to Your will. Thank you for giving me the tools I need to defeat the enemy. I give You all the praise for the victory I know is coming in Your name.*

I HAVE TO PRACTICE
WHAT I PREACH

On December 4, 2011 I was running in a ravine that was lined with big limestone rocks. I decided it would be fun to do agility drills, running side to side up and down the length of the ravine. I continued doing this for about 45 minutes, feeling like Superwoman. As I jumped out to the last rock, my ankle gave way. It popped with a sound like a stick being snapped in two, and I knew it must be broken.

I know God's Word so I grabbed my leg and I prayed, "Lord, I know that this is not your will. I know the enemy comes to steal, kill and destroy, but you have come to give me abundant life. Search my heart, God. If there is anything that I need to repent of, show me right now." Our heavenly Father is so faithful. Right in that moment, He illuminated a spirit of pride that I needed to deal with. The rock that I was laying on became my altar of sacrifice as I laid my sin out there and asked for forgiveness. I fully repented for my pride and arrogance. I also asked the Father for supernatural healing because I was walking down the aisle to marry the most wonderful man I had ever known in 23 days and then we were off to Kauai for a ten-day adventure honeymoon.

An elderly couple passing by came to help me off the rock. We were quite the sight getting back up that ravine. My fiancé came as fast as he could to pick me up and we went to the emergency room. Things were not

looking good. My ankle was swelling and turning pur-
ple and black—but I had no pain. They took X-rays and
told me that it was not broken, but it was a severe high
ankle sprain and that it would probably take longer than
a break to heal because of the severity of the injury. As an
active personal trainer with an upcoming wedding, this
was not the news I wanted to hear.

We left the hospital, picked up the pain medications and crutches, and my fiancé took me home. After
he had propped me up and headed home, I just had to
pray, "God, this is a pretty hard thing, but I know that
You are working in the unseen and I trust that You will
be faithful to heal me." I trusted God he would provide
supernatural healing and that I wouldn't have to relay on
the Hydrocodon that was prescribed for pain. I never had
to take a single pill. Now that bottle serves as a reminder
that my God was so faithful!

Six days later, I was hobbling around on crutches,
attempting to put out my nativity set. I was having a time
of worship and singing to God as I was laying Baby Jesus
in the little manger. At that moment, I heard the Lord
say, "Take a step of faith." I knew that God was asking me
to lay down my crutches and test my faith. Some people
would say that was ridiculous, but I know the God that I
serve and I knew He was asking me to do something, so I
obeyed. I laid down the crutches and I walked. I had to be
gentle, but I did it! I never picked up the crutches again. I
walked barefoot down the aisle in a historic prairie church
to marry my wonderful, godly husband! We went on our
honeymoon and instead of the fast-paced adventure we
had planned, God allowed us to lie on the beach, read and
worship together, have picnics, relax, and be refreshed.

Most people who know me understand that relaxing and being still is not something that I really enjoy. It's not in my nature. I prefer to keep busy. I will admit that before the Fit for Freedom Challenge, I often had been tempted to take on too many things because I was too driven. During the Challenge, I was managing a huge group of 175 people and ministering to their needs through prayer, teaching, emails and phone calls, personal meetings and more. Two weeks into the Challenge, I took what was already a great idea and started adding more and more to it, making more work for myself and creating needless stress on my body.

At this point, I was still healing from my ankle injury and I wasn't able to exercise at my usual level. I had taken on needless stress by adding more components to the Challenge and that was causing me to have to stay up way past my bedtime. I wasn't eating properly either, in fact, I was so busy I was forgetting to eat. Without enough exercise, getting very little sleep, and eating too little and not making the best choices in my hurried days, the inevitable happened—while everybody else was *Losing IT*, I was gaining it!

Two months into the program, God showed me something profound. Several years ago, I had allowed myself to become wrapped up in performance because of something that one of my ex-husband's relatives had said to me. This person told me that I had never been anything, I never would be anything, and if it weren't for my former husband I would never have had anything to call my own. I was hurt. I knew this wasn't true and that they were speaking to me out of their own pain over the situation. I thought I had dismissed it, but unconsciously I began to strive for success to make sure that everyone knew that comment about me was wrong. Instead of relying on God to be my source and combating those words spoken over me with His truths, I chose to take the burden upon myself.

As a single mom, I had strived, worked and pressed forward—for my own glory. I hate to admit it, but instead of giving glory to God for all He had miraculously given me, I started becoming prideful. In my heart, I was saying, "Yay me! I work with the Biggest Losers. Look at all the important people I know. Look at all the people who think I'm really good at what I do."

The Bible says that "pride goeth before a fall." I am so thankful that the God of mercy illuminated my pride to me that day that I was sitting on the rock holding my ankle. In my case, the fall came before I was aware of how prideful I was. But once He showed me my sin and I repented of it, God was able to move quickly on my behalf.

A few weeks later, near the end of the Challenge, I was absolutely exhausted. I know God called us to do hard things for Him, but He promises not to give us more than we can handle. I had made my tasks harder than He intended by trying to do things my own way. God showed me my driven nature, and how my behavior was robbing me of good health. He shined His big flashlight on the fact that I was creating unnecessary anxiety and stress by adding too many projects on top of what was already a great plan from Him. I once again had the opportunity to repent and turn myself around and LIVE (Ezekiel 18:32). I had a choice, and I chose to let go and to receive God's rest, not just for the duration of the Challenge, but for the weeks and months after it ended.

NOW WHAT?

Now that you've finished this wellness devotional, you may be asking yourself, "Where do I go from here?" I want you to understand that there are some very important keys that I have given to you that will determine your success or failure when it comes to your health. Please meditate on these truths and let them penetrate your heart.

First of all, you must realize that the enemy is very strategic about using two particularly effective weapons to destroy your success and take back the ground you have gained. The first weapon Satan uses is your thoughts. He will bring every kind of lie and accusation to your mind to defeat you and throw you headlong off your course to health and wellness. 2 Corinthians 10:5 says that you must "cast down imaginations, and every high thing that exalts itself against the knowledge of God, and bring into captivity every thought to the obedience of Christ." How do you do that? By using your most potent weapon—the sword of the Spirit. Hebrews 4:12 tells us that "the word of God is living and active and sharper than any two-edged sword." When the enemy comes you MUST have a storehouse of scriptures that you can pull out and use to fight him off.

The second weapon that the devil uses is your own words. He very slyly gets you to repeat words from your past vocabulary over your life. He uses those words as seeds to plant in the fertile soil of your heart. He wants you to believe that you are never going to have a healthy body, that you will never be able to lose weight, that you are always going to be a nobody, that you are too weak to exercise consistently, and that you are generally worthless. He often starts with a negative thought or negative words spoken over you from the past, then has you meditate on them if you don't quickly cast those thoughts down. Once the negative thoughts and words drop into your heart, they become a part of you. Pretty soon, you are speaking that negativity out of your own mouth. The Bible says that "out of the abundance of the heart the mouth speaks." I want the abundance of my heart to speak blessings over my health and my body. Matthew 12:37 says, "For by your words you shall be justified, and by your words you shall be condemned." Positive, uplifting words produce faith and negative words bring condemnation. Choose carefully what you let into your mind, for those same words will soon come out of your mouth.

Recently, I had to deal with this in my own life. I have been walking towards my healing for almost ten years now. I have overcome addictions, self-defeating emotions, and unforgiveness in order to move forward and hold on to my healing. But the enemy is always watching for an opportunity to come back into my life to try to trip me up again, he's always looking for the slightest crack. I'll share with you the latest chapter in my struggle with negative thoughts.

On the day after Thanksgiving, my husband and I decided to take our children for an overnight vacation to a fancy hotel in town. They have a huge Christmas display and we thought that it would be a fun way to bond since we are not really into Black Friday shopping. There were hundreds of people milling about, checking out the displays. As we walked around, I began to notice all these tall, beautiful women in stretchy riding jeans and high-heeled boots. Now, Satan knows that I have always had a struggle with my legs. They are thick and athletic, and no matter how hard I work on them, they do not get super lean. I've come to accept it and make what I have as tight as possible, but for the most part I don't obsess about my legs anymore.

However, on this day, everywhere we went, I saw these ladies with their beautiful, thin legs! I started listening to Satan's condemning thoughts. "Well, you really shouldn't have had that pumpkin pie yesterday. No wonder your legs are so big. You are never going to have legs like theirs. You look so gross. You should have dressed up more. You'll never look as good as they do. You have gained 12 pounds since your ankle injury. You are so fat." Believe it or not, I felt myself accepting these lies and I literally felt depression sweep over me. I wanted to run to my room and be alone.

I knew what I had to do. I started saying in my mind, "I rebuke your thoughts, Satan. Those thoughts are not who I am. Christ says I am a masterpiece created unto Him to do good works. God calls me loved. God calls me beautiful and chosen." I brought to mind scriptures that I have in my arsenal and told the enemy that I would not receive his lies. Furthermore, rather than suffering in silence, when we got to our room at the end of the even-ing I told my husband about the battle that had been taking place in my mind. We came together in agreement and he gently laid hands on me and commanded the tormenting thoughts to leave. Helpless in the power of our united prayer, the devil tucked his tail and ran. All the negative thoughts left. The next day I had a good laugh when we went down to breakfast and noticed all the same ladies looking as average in their sweats as I did in mine!

I've said it once, and I'll say it again—you will succeed or fail by the thoughts that you think and the words that you speak.

LAURIE'S WELLNESS TIPS

Here are my top tips that will keep you on the road to wellness:

1. You need accountability! Find a friend, start a support group, join a weight loss group at your church—whatever you need to do to be accountable to someone with your decision to get healthy. It's the number one key to sticking with your plan.
2. Write down what you eat. Most people have no idea of how much or how often they are consuming food. I have used a food journal for years. It keeps me on track and helps me be accountable and realistic about what I'm eating. There are apps for your smartphone that make this a really easy process. For me, there is just something about the act of writing it down, so I have a journal that I keep in my kitchen and put it in my purse when I leave the house or take a vacation. I write in it every day and I also record my exercise there too.
3. If you are struggling with knowing what to eat, don't stress or worry about it. Start slowly with the foods that are reasonable for you and your lifestyle. You do not have to completely change your diet all at once. In fact, if you do, you may become completely overwhelmed and give up before you have time to see the plan actually work.

Make small realistic changes every week and by the end of the year those 52 little changes will add up to inches off your waist! Here are some simple guidelines for choosing healthy foods:

- Choose lean protein such as fish, turkey, chicken or lean cuts of beef.
- Mom was right—eat your veggies and fruits. Eat all the colors of the rainbow.
- Choose low-fat dairy products and enjoy cheese and butter in moderation.
- Eat plenty of fiber and whole grains like brown rice, 100% whole wheat bread, corn tortillas and oatmeal. Many people cut out carbohydrates completely when dieting, but this can be counter-productive since carbs help support brain function and energy for movement. One tip that is helpful when trying to lose weight is to limit carbohydrates to the breakfast and lunch meals and have lean protein and vegetables for your evening meal.
- Try to limit the number of times you go out to eat. Restaurant meals tend to be high in fat and salt even if you are picking the healthiest items on the menu.
- Eat a salad with lunch and dinner. Try to fill half of your plate with salad or vegetables (corn and potatoes are not vegetables), one quarter with a complex carbohydrate such as brown rice, whole wheat pasta, or yellow squash and one quarter with your lean meat choice for a balanced meal.

- Use a smaller plate. It will trick your eye and brain into thinking you've eaten more that you actually have.

  If you need additional nutritional information, you can find it at a bookstore or your local library. There are many books that outline a healthy eating plan.

4. Get some exercise. It's a must. Exercise gets the blood flowing, it helps your body shake off stress and anxiety, and it wards off depression. Weight-bearing exercise helps your joints and bones stay strong as you age. Aerobic exercise such as walking, jogging, swimming and bicycling helps your heart stay healthy and your body stay thinner. My best advice is to pick something you liked to do as a kid and try that first. If you aren't sure what to do, try walking. Most people can do it, and the only equipment you need is a good pair of athletic shoes. Try to exercise at least 2-3 times per week for thirty minutes. Some individuals may have to begin with less than thirty minutes, but you can build up your level of fitness if you are consistent. If you are not sure how to properly use the equipment at the gym, do yourself a favor and invest in a few personal training sessions to get you started on the right track and prevent injury.

5. Drink your water. After a long night's sleep with your mouth open and drawing in air, you become dehydrated. Start the day off right with sixteen ounces of water. It will help jumpstart your metabolism for the day. And remember to keep

drinking water all day long. Many times our body can mistake thirst as hunger. If you have eaten recently and feel hungry, try drinking a big glass of water. It you still feel legitimately hungry, have a healthy snack such as a piece of fruit, low-fat yogurt or a small handful of almonds.

6. Sleep is vital to your weight loss and wellness success. When you don't get between seven and eight hours of sleep per night, your body goes into overdrive, producing too much cortisol which in turn causes you to gain belly fat. I hear many people say, "I only need four or five hours of sleep." Actually, you need the same amount of sleep as the rest of us. You've just trained yourself to make do with less. Unfortunately, this habit is devastating to your immune system. Without enough rest, your cells don't regenerate the way they are supposed to, your brain can't function properly, and all of your organs have to work harder to support the damage you are doing nightly by not getting enough sleep.

If you are having a difficult time falling asleep, try these tips:

- Sleep in a totally dark room.
- Remove electronics and LED lights of any kind. Even the subtle light from your bedside alarm clock can prevent you from falling into a deep sleep.
- Sleep in a cool room with the thermostat set to 70 degrees or less.

- Try not to eat two to three hours before bedtime.
- Read God's Word before bed. It brings peace.
- Thank God for all the blessings He has given you this day.
- Remember to pray and confess so that your mind is at ease and sweet sleep can come.

7. Finally, remember that you must allow the Holy Spirit to speak to you about what is right for *your* body. Because everyone is different, every journey to physical fitness is different. Your journey may take longer or it may be shorter than your friend's. God may give you a plan that is right for the first three months, but then you may find He asks you to make adjustments to it for the next three months. Whatever your plan, do not listen to all of the hype for quick weight loss. It is not realistic or sustainable. Pills, extreme diets and weird exercise gadgets do not work, but the power of the Holy Spirit does. He will guide you and He will lead you to a fit, energetic body in His timing and according to His plan.

Some of you may be saying, "I've read the book, but I don't know if I have the relationship with God that's required to begin this spiritual journey to wellness." There is a very simple way to fix that. Pray this prayer with me now:

Dear Jesus, I know I am lost without You. I've been trying to make my life work without You and I realize now that I need your help. I choose today to follow

You and invite You into my life. Jesus, I confess You are the Son of God and that You died for my sins. I receive your grace and freedom and release my old life, my sins, and my addictions and ask you to exchange all of that for the new life You have promised me in Your word. I thank You that I am Your child now and that You will teach me and lead me from this day forward. Amen.

If you prayed that prayer for the first time, congratulations! You are now a daughter or son of the Most High God.

I bless all of you who have taken the time to read these devotionals and apply these principles to your life. May you be empowered to receive God's healing of your spirit, soul, and body. I declare that in Jesus's name all of God's plans for you are good. You are equipped and able to take back what the enemy has tried to steal from you. I proclaim by faith that you will receive healing, weight loss, smaller sizes, energy and confidence to move out and become all that God has called you to be! Go now in good health!

ABOUT FAMILY LEGACY MISSIONS INTERNATIONAL

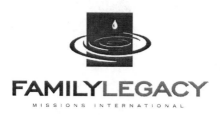

A portion of proceeds from *Fit for Freedom* will benefit the Family Legacy Missions International.

In June of 2000, Greer Kendall traveled back to the country of his birth–Zambia, Africa–for the first time since he left as a six-year-old boy. It was a trip that changed everything. Returning again in July and then in September with his wife, Susan, the Lord began to open Greer's eyes to the stark and shocking reality of the orphan crisis in this south central African country.

Due to the scourge of HIV/AIDS and the extreme poverty that breeds hopelessness and despair, Zambia had become home to the largest percentage of orphans in any country in the world. Over one million orphaned children in a land of only 12 million. Zambia was a land in crisis, on the brink of destruction, and the children were quickly becoming a lost and abandoned generation.

The Lord led Greer to incorporate Family Legacy Missions International in September of 2000. Since that time, the Kendall family, including children Jonathan, Karis, and Kaleigh, and the staff of Family Legacy have committed to one goal: transforming Zambia one child at a time.

Family Legacy Missions International exists to connect American families with the orphans and vulnerable children of Zambia to proclaim the gospel, transform lives, and rescue orphans. This organization focuses on three main ministries: Camp LIFE, Father's Heart, and Tree of Life.

Camp LIFE brings together American volunteers to engage in the call of the Great Commission. While at camp, these children learn how much God loves them through their camp counselors. Through one-on-one time, Americans learn more about each child's family life and prayer needs. During these special times of blessing, many children find a safe place to open up about the difficult situations they face and find freedom and healing through the love of Jesus Christ.

The Father's Heart Sponsorship Program allows individuals and families to sponsor children and provide for the child's ongoing needs, including discipleship and education. Through this program, children who are sponsored are able to attend a quality school and receive the support of Zambian pastors and chaplains, as well as field workers who build relationships with the children and families.

Family Legacy's LIFEWAY Christian Academies (LCAs) are the centerpiece of the Father's Heart program. The LIFEWAY Christian Academies provide a private, Christian education to our sponsored children in grades 1-6. LCAs are marked by high-quality teachers, low student-to-teacher ratios, on-going teacher training, and an education that truly prepares these children for the future. Children also benefit from nutrient and protein-rich daily school lunches to ensure they are physically nourished.

The Tree of Life Children's Village, located just outside the capital city of Lusaka, is a 130-acre community of homes for orphaned children designed to be a haven of hope and light. The organization's vision is to build twelve Children's Villages throughout the country of Zambia to rescue orphans from abuse and poverty and bring holistic change to a nation in need. Children at the Tree of Life receive both educational and spiritual development that will dramatically transform their future. Full-time pastors build on this by teaching the Word of God and encouraging the children in their faith.

Through their three crucial ministries to the orphans and vulnerable children of Zambia, Family Legacy Missions International is seeing transformation happen daily in the lives of thousands of children. It is these very children who are the future of Zambia – the ones whose lives will ripple in impact for generations to come and who will bring lasting transformation to the country they call home.

To learn more, please visit our website:
www.familylegacy.com.

ABOUT THE AUTHOR

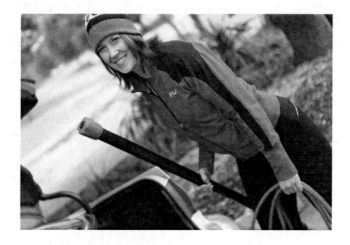

Laurie is able to relate to her obese clients. As a teenager she suffered with anorexia and bulimia. Through her 20s and early 30s, she medicated the pain of life with food. Nine years ago, she was 90 pounds overweight and clinically depressed. Then a personal trainer put a flyer on her door that changed everything. She decided to get fit and ended up having a total physical transformation. She went on to become a figure and fitness competitor and completely changed her outer appearance. Inside, however, her spirit and soul continued to suffer because she had not addressed the root of the food addiction and other painful issues in her life.

In 2009, she experienced a spiritual breakthrough when she realized that her worth was not based on the way her body looked, but on her identity in Christ. In 2010, she led her first spiritual accountability and exercise group for women at Prestonwood Baptist Church in Plano, TX. Today, she inspires women's groups and entire congregations with faith and fitness leadership and has taught hundreds of people how to live healthier and happier lives. She is also involved in a youth ministry with her teenage daughter at a Section 8 apartment complex in her community and is involved with a multi-faith women's fellowship group, *Embrace.*

Laurie is a National Academy of Sports Medicine certified personal trainer. As an independent trainer, she trains and mentors contestants and former contestants from NBC's *The Biggest Loser* and ABC's *Extreme Weight Loss* in her local area, as well as stay-at-home moms, students, dancers, actors, and business executives. She also inspires women's groups and entire congregations with faith and fitness leadership. She has taught hundreds of people how to live healthier and happier lives. Laurie is successful in helping people achieve their weight loss goals. She aids them in learning effective ways to maintain a healthy lifestyle through proven biblical principles of the body, soul, and spirit.

Some of her notable training and mentoring clients include:

- Earl Kennedy, a former 913-pound man
- Renee Wilson, former contestant on *The Biggest Loser*, season 6
- Sandy Dolan, at-home contestant on *The Biggest Loser*, season 10

- Aaron Thompkins, former contestant on *The Biggest Loser*, season 10
- Staci Birdwell, former star on *Extreme Extreme Weight Loss Edition*, season 1
- Brian Justin Crum, Broadway actor/dancer, *Grease, Tarzan,* and starring as Daniel Brooks in *"Law and Order: Special Victims Unit" Possessed* (TV episode 2011)

Laurie has been featured in articles in the Fort Worth Star Telegram and The Keller Citizen. Stories with her clients have been aired on NBC 5 Dallas and NBC 10 Oklahoma. She lives in Texas with her husband and children.

For more information about Laurie's training and ministry, how Laurie can help you with virtual coaching and mentoring programs, to contact her about a speaking at an upcoming event in your community or at your church, and to see the ways she's impacting the health and wellness industry for Christ…visit *www.lauriegraves.com.*

To learn more about exercise and nutritional products Laurie has to offer as an Independent Team Beachbody® Coach and Shakeology® ditributor, visit *www.lauriefit.com.*

FIT FOR FREEDOM
faithandfitness.net/**freedom** ⏻*NLINE*

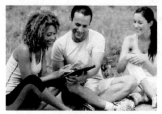

Stay Motivated with your FREE online tools and resources.

+ Healthy Eating Guide
+ Printable resources for individuals and groups
+ Easy-to-use Spiritual strengthening tools
+ Positive Changes Guide
+ Laurie's latest BLOG postings
+ Events
+ Access to additional content

You have the book. Now visit faithandfitness.net/freedom to stay FIT FOR FREEDOM.